NML/FF

Please return / renew by date shown.
You can renew at: **norlink.norfolk.gov.uk**
or by telephone: **0344 800 8006**
Please have your library card & PIN ready.

NORFOLK LIBRARY
AND INFORMATION SERVICE

dedication

This book is dedicated to all the babies, mothers, fathers and families that I
have had the honour of being with during their birth journeys, and to everyone
I have worked alongside in the 'maternity NHS family', my second home. I would
also like to dedicate this book to all those that support the NHS on the outer circle,
such as the wonderful doulas and complementary therapists that help
mothers have a healthy and positive birth experience.

your body
your baby
your birth

the must-have handbook to help you have
the best possible pregnancy, labour and birth

Jenny Smith

with Charlotte Edwardes

RODALE

This edition first published 2009 by Rodale
an imprint of Pan Macmillan Ltd
Pan Macmillan, 20 New Wharf Road, London N1 9RR
Basingstoke and Oxford
Associated companies throughout the world
www.panmacmillan.com

ISBN 978-1-9057-44-31-2

1 3 5 7 9 8 6 4 2

A CIP catalogue record for this book is available from the British Library.

Editorial director: Liz Gough
Editor: Salima Hirani
Assistant editor: Anya Wilson
Proofreader: Charlotte Ridings
Indexer: Hilary Bird
Jacket design: Katie Tooke
Page design, typesetting and illustrations: Simon Daley

Printed and bound in the UK by CPI Mackays, Chatham ME5 8TD

All photographs © Getty Images

This book is intended as a reference volume only, not as a medical manual. The information given
here is designed to help you make informed decisions about your health. It is not intended as a substitute
for any treatment that you may have been prescribed by your doctor. If you suspect you have a medical
problem, we urge you to seek competent medical help.
Mention of specific companies, organizations or authorities in this book does not imply endorsement of the publisher,
nor does mention of specific companies, organizations or authorities in the book imply that they endorse the book.

Addresses, websites and telephone numbers given in this book were correct at the time of going to press.

Visit **www.panmacmillan.com** to read more about all our books and to buy them. You will also find features,
author interviews and news of any author events, and you can sign up for e-newsletters so that you're
always first to hear about our new releases.

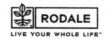

We inspire and enable people to improve their lives and the world around them

contents

acknowledgements

First and foremost, I would like to thank each and every mother, father and baby for whom I have had the honour of being their midwife.

Importantly, I would like to express my deepest gratitude to Charlotte Edwardes who made the book a reality and to the most fabulous team of Elizabeth Sheinkman, my agent at Curtis Brown, Liz Gough, Editorial Director Rodale UK, editor Salima Hirani and designer Simon Daley. Sincere thanks are also due to Gabby Logan and Michel Odent for their kind endorsements.

I am also indebted to everyone at Queen Charlotte's and Chelsea Hospital for always making me feel part of the family. I would especially like to thank Jackie Fox, and Wendy Lane who makes me smile every morning.

Each of the following people have provided valuable support and guidance over the years: Mr Edmonds, CPG Director; Ms Maggie O'Brien, Director of Midwifery and Nursing; Mr Kumar; Mr McCarthy; Ms Stalder and all in the obstetric anaesthetic and neonatal consultant teams; Valda Armstrong (for always being there – my soul mate in midwifery); Verna Springer; Ann Maloy; Abigail Snow; Graham Pajak; Alpa Patel; Simi Ojelade; Candida Rom; Joan Glasgow; Stephanie Greenaway; Dr Vasso Teridou; Dr Lucy Chappell; Professor Bennett (for his constant support – I consider him to be an honorary midwife); Sara Paterson-Brown (an obstetric champion); Ruwan Wimalasundera (for his reassurance and sensible advice); Felicity Plaat (for her ability to see pain relief in all its dimensions); Mandish Dhanjal (for her normality focus); and Professor Fisk (for his wisdom).

I would also like to thank my own obstetrician Dr Fergusson, who has influenced my practice throughout the years and my own special midwives Francine Allen, Evelyn Jackson and Helen Ross-McGill, all of whom I consider to be part of my family.

A huge thank you is due to Michel Odent, a global pioneer, and Gowri Motha, Nel Linsdell, Nicki O'Clarey and Ramona Peoples, all of whom have expanded my horizons. Also to Marika Salzer (Global Marketing, Philips), Mark Peacock (Cardiac Services), Ruth Meadows, for her support in the changing journey, Mary Wrigley, Sally Ashton-May and Rixa Von dem Bussche. I also wish to thank Nick Samuels, Jan Preece , Charlotte Mayou, Dee Ward, Adam Lamb, Ben Cowlin and my dear personal friends doctors Sally and Mark Tattersall, Gena and Nick Wright, Penny Hocknell and Lucy and Patrick Woodroffe.

Forever, I will be deeply grateful to my committee for taking a leap of faith and establishing The Jentle Childbirth Foundation.

Finally, from the bottom of my heart, a huge thank you to my own family: Ed, Oliver, Emma, Oscar and Elizabeth, and my parents Joan and Jim, for their understanding and embracing of my passion for midwifery and for generously accommodating all that it entails in their lives.

foreword BY PROFESSOR PHILLIP BENNETT

Most of our ancestors were born at home, helped into the world by the highly experienced local midwife or, as we go further back in history, a grandmother, aunt, wise friend or relation. There was no formal antenatal care. Women knew what to expect in their pregnancy from the experience of women around them, whose collective knowledge of pregnancy, labour and delivery was substantial. In the 20th century important developments such as antibiotic therapy and blood transfusion made childbirth safer, but had the unfortunate side effect of making pregnancy seem like a disease. Antenatal care became focused on hospital-based consultant-lead units and, increasingly, labour and delivery took place, not at home, but in the hospital. The introduction of electronic fetal heart-rate monitoring in labour in the late 1960s lead to almost every baby being a hospital birth, and to the near extinction of the experienced community midwife.

'Jenny Smith has helped to break down the barriers between natural childbirth and medical care. She is a midwife who strives to make every childbirth as normal, stress free and fulfilling as possible.'

I delivered my first baby as a medical student in 1980, in a brightly lit delivery room, with the mother's legs in stirrups and covered by surgical drapes. Both myself and the midwife who was teaching me were wearing green sterile gowns, hats, masks and gloves. We had a big tray of instruments in our delivery pack with lots of swabs and towels. It was more like a surgical operation than a natural event. But that first experience of a baby being born had a profound effect upon me, and was one of the reasons why I decided to become an obstetrician.

In the last two decades we have seen a reversal of this medicalization of childbirth. A minority of women do develop serious illness during pregnancy and, for these few, care in an obviously medical environment is essential, but for the majority of women we have now done away with the sterile gowns, hats and masks, and with the stirrups, and instead have rooms with hidden medical equipment, low lighting and comfortable beds. Babies are delivered on the bed, on the floor, on a bean bag or a birthing stool, and even sometimes underwater. Increasingly, antenatal care in uncomplicated pregnancies is focusing back upon one-to-one or community midwifery teams and, gradually, we are returning to home births for women at low risk and who want to do that.

But in parallel with the reversal of the medicalization of childbirth we have seen an increase in our ability to look into the womb and predict problems for the unborn child, which has pushed pregnancy back onto the medical stage. Although less than 1% of babies have serious problems, this ability can lead to great anxiety, which can be heightened by that great 21st century phenomenon, the internet, which dispenses unregulated, unrestricted and frequently conflicting advice from anybody who has an angle and owns a computer.

Pregnancy and childbirth are very special times for a family, but they are also times of anxiety and risk. The modern obstetrician and midwife must play two roles: supporter, friend and counsellor when things go normally; and medical carer when there are problems. I have worked with Jenny Smith for several years. I often say to couples who see me for the first time in their pregnancy that I will help them to have their baby in any way that they want to, provided that it is safe. But I think that Jenny has a more extended philosophy; that we should all strive to make childbirth as fulfilling an experience as possible, no matter how it eventually happens. Jenny's philosophy is that every woman needs to be fully prepared for childbirth. Understanding what will happen and why it will happen reduces anxiety and makes things go much more smoothly. Jenny has helped to break down the barriers between natural childbirth and medical care. She has shown, for example, that induction of labour and a waterbirth are not incompatible, that skin-to-skin contact between mother and baby can occur just as quickly and easily when birth is by Caesarean as when it is normal, and that everybody, not just those planning an intervention-free labour, can benefit from good advice and proper preparation.

In the last decade or so, with the development of team and one-to-one midwifery, I have seen a much greater degree of integration and co-operation between obstetricians and midwives. Both have their role to play and they need to work together in harmony to ensure the best outcomes. Jenny Smith is a midwife at the forefront of this movement, a midwife who strives to make every childbirth as normal, stress free and fulfilling as possible. This book is a distillation of her philosophy. The information in it should help every pregnant woman and her family understand the changes which will happen in her body, the checks and tests that will happen during the pregnancy, and to prepare for the big day when she meets her new baby for the first time.

PROFESSOR PHILLIP BENNETT BSC PHD MD FRCOG, CONSULTANT OBSTETRICIAN
QUEEN CHARLOTTE'S AND CHELSEA HOSPITAL, LONDON AND IMPERIAL COLLEGE, LONDON.

introduction

I always say that a first-time mother is a completely different species to a second-time mother. With the benefit of experience, the latter is more prepared, both mentally and physiologically, for labour and birth. But I know that a first-time mother can also feel prepared – prepared enough to be able to greatly increase her chances of a 'normal' (vaginal), relatively stress-free, even peaceful, birth. If there is one thing that I have learned in over a quarter of a century as a midwife, it is that *all* births can be positive (whatever way the baby is born). For an expectant mother, preparation is the key.

There are many ways in which you can make your birth experience a positive one, and my aim is to show you how, by making this book the literary equivalent of having your own one-to-one midwife. One of my central beliefs is that a pregnant woman cannot expect the professionals to do everything – particularly when she is in the care of the NHS. You have to help yourself. You need to make decisions for yourself and be willing to participate. You cannot play a passive role if you want a positive outcome. I have learned that first-time mothers *are* able to trust in their bodies, their instincts and their own decisions, if only they know how. In this book, I hope to guide you towards that knowledge.

In part one, I start by helping you enjoy your pregnancy as much as you can, to take care of and connect with the new life growing within you, and I offer tips on how to cope with the physical changes of pregnancy and deal with the practicalities of taking care of yourself in a busy life. I will also guide you through the maze of antenatal care during each trimester, providing information on your rights and choices so you can make the most of the care on offer to you. And I will help you prepare for parenthood, talking through the important issues that concern taking responsibility for your wonderful new baby.

During pregnancy is the best time to prepare for the birth. In part two, I discuss in detail the choices available on the NHS for birth (many of which you may not even know you have), explain what you can expect from your care providers during the birth, what you are entitled to, and prompt you with a series of questions to ask yourself, your birth partner and your care providers to help you decide what kind of birth you want and find out how best to achieve it. I provide information on all the options for pain relief – both natural methods and in the form of drugs. And I pass on the expertise I have developed during my career that can help make the birth proceed as smoothly as possible.

One of my strongest beliefs is that the mental strength to get through labour is inbuilt in all women. Most women fear childbirth, but you have the power to overcome your fears and even enjoy the experience! You just need to learn the techniques and do the training so that you feel completely prepared. In this book I will help you to train and harness the power of your mind. I call this 'making the head stronger than the uterus', by which I mean developing the mental strength to cope with each contraction as it comes. If there is one thing I hear myself saying more than anything at work, it's 'You can do it!', and trust me, *you* can. You just need to tap into that strength and make it work for you.

I have what I call a 'tool box' of ideas you can choose from to help you do this. One of these tools is visualisation. I have witnessed first-hand incredible outcomes for women who have simply trained their minds to overcome quite staggering odds. In this book I show you how to develop a tailor-made visualisation you can turn to to help you through your labour. I explain how and when to use complementary therapies such as reflexology and aromatherapy during pregnancy and labour, how to use visual aids and develop rituals to help you focus your mind during each contraction, how to use powerful breathing exercises to manage pain and keep you calm, and suggest how to select your own 'snuggly bits', as I call them, which are those comforting personal items that can help you relax and feel confident during labour and birth. Most importantly, I will help you to have faith in yourself and your own abilities, which is your greatest tool for achieving the most positive birth experience.

Even if yours is a 'high-risk' pregnancy, or if things don't turn out during the birth as you had planned during labour and birth, there is much you can do to maintain control of the events and still enjoy it. In almost any birth situation 'natural' and 'normal' elements can be introduced. I want to challenge the norm of insisting that 'high-risk' women lie on a bed for birth, attached to a fetal heart monitor, surrounded by drip stands, with anxious father-to-be and concerned attendants at the bedside. It's not necessary. With the advent of Telemetry (remote monitoring), women in high-risk situations can use the equipment of low-tech births, such as birthing pools, bean bags, birthing stools and so on.

In part three of this book, I will guide you through the first six weeks of caring for your newborn baby, helping you navigate this special but also very challenging time and focus on what is important for you and your family.

THE 'JENTLE' LANGUAGE

Most women in the UK give birth on mainstream NHS labour wards. Simple things, such as kindness, empathy, respect, flexibility and patience can sometimes get forgotten on busy maternity wards. But these things – I am not exaggerating – can determine a positive or negative birth experience, and the life-long consequences that go with that. Labouring women should not be looked down on, they should be met eye-to-eye, allowed to move about and sit on rocking chairs (with monitors attached if necessary). They should be allowed to enjoy music and dimmed lighting if they want, helped to feel comfortable, and able to have their say in how things should proceed. I have seen for myself how labouring mothers, comforted in this way, do much better during childbirth than those that feel uncomfortable, unimportant or ignored. Even the most medicalized birth can be a very positive experience for a mother who feels empowered in the situation and has the aid of small but important comforts.

I realised a long time ago that what women want from a midwife to help them feel comfortable and confident is continuity of communication, privacy, trust, kindness, understanding, compassion, being listened to and understood. I learned to base my approach as a midwife on meeting these needs, and was fortunate enough to run the Jentle Scheme of Midwifery at Queen Charlotte's and Chelsea Hospital between 2004 and 2007. This highly successful scheme was born out of a passionate belief shared between myself and the mothers in my care – that each woman can have a positive birth experience.

With the support of highly collaborative senior obstetricians, I worked with hundreds of women to help them achieve the kind of births they wanted, and also brought many high-risk women into the gentle surroundings commonly associated with 'natural' birth. I provided one-to-one midwifery care, helped women understand the birthing process, worked with them to devise a personal 'Utopia birth plan' and prepare for the unexpected (to enable them to reclaim their births even when things didn't go according to plan) and, most importantly, listened to their needs and tried to meet them. 'Jentle' became like a new language of midwifery that I shared with the women in my care.

Many of my women asked me to write down all that I shared with them on our journey to birth, so this book is the heritage of the Jentle Scheme of Midwifery. I hope it helps you prepare for one of the biggest events you will experience in your life, and that you enjoy every moment of it.

JENNY SMITH, FEBRUARY 2009

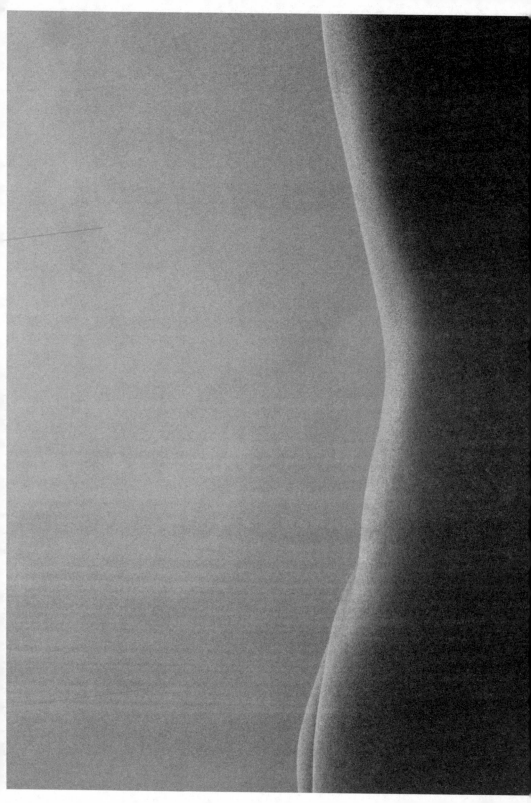

PART ONE

your pregnancy

first trimester 0–12 weeks

This is an extraordinary time: you have just discovered you are pregnant and a new life has begun. You are embarking on a wonderful journey during which this new life will steadily grow into the little baby that you and your partner will hold in your arms. This journey will take you both through the most incredible range of feelings, mentally and physically. It will not always be easy. The more knowledge you have about what is happening to you, the more empowered and prepared you will feel. Whatever your pregnancy throws you, try to stay positive.

am I really pregnant?

Most women who are trying to conceive find the two weeks after ovulation an agonizing wait. Some say they noticed early symptoms – such as sore breasts, increased discharge or 'implantation bleeding' – not long after conception.

Common signs of pregnancy are listed on pages 17–29. Don't worry if you don't have all of the symptoms – some women don't get any.

The next step is to take a pregnancy test. You can buy a home pregnancy test from a pharmacy or get one for free from a family planning clinic. Follow the instructions carefully. The cost varies between seven and ten pounds and will give you a quick, hassle-free result.

Pregnancy tests detect the level of human Chorionic Gonadotropin (hCG) hormone in your urine and some home tests are sensitive enough to pick up this early pregnancy hormone a few days before your expected period. I've heard of women, desperately trying to get pregnant, who spend a fortune on tests every month, and test right up until the dreaded moment their period arrives. It's best to wait until you miss your period to test, as you may have a negative result purely because the level of hCG is still too low for the test to detect.

If you wait until you have missed your period before you test, it will be 97% accurate. If you don't get your period, the test is negative, but you still think you may be pregnant, see your GP.

what do I do now?

If you haven't already, a good next step is to make an appointment with the GP. This is sensible for a number of reasons. The GP will:

- ⊙ test your urine
- ⊙ check your blood pressure (this provides a baseline of your normal blood pressure to check against later in pregnancy – high blood pressure when pregnant can cause serious problems
- ⊙ check your height and weight (your GP may comment on your body mass index, or BMI (see pages 64–5) – particularly if you are underweight or overweight)

- recommend that, if you haven't already, you take folic acid tablets. If you are on a low income, you can get help from Healthy Start (see page 328 for contact details), the government initiative that provides free vitamins and vouchers to buy cows' milk, fresh fruit and vegetables
- ask you for your medical history. Mention anything you think is important, for example, if you know that you are rhesus negative
- refer you to the local hospital. Make sure your GP's letter includes your medical and obstetric history in full. It may be that a particular hospital has the specialized services you require.

The last point is essential: your GP is your gateway to maternity services. In future the government hope to introduce midwives linked to GPs' practices who will be responsible for initial tests and referrals.

Within the NHS there is also a system of 'shared care', which means you can see your GP for 50% (or more) of your antenatal appointments, with the remainder being undertaken at the hospital.

when can I tell everyone my exciting news?

Many women wait until they have weathered the first 12 weeks, and the most precarious trimester, before announcing their pregnancies. The risk of miscarriage is great in the early weeks so most people delay the announcement until they have been scanned and given the all clear by the hospital.

Obviously the urge to tell is great, and women do confide in close family and friends – as well as a few random people they will never see again, such as the woman sitting next to you on the train, or a shop assistant.

There may also be a need to tell your boss, particularly if you are feeling very unwell and need time off, or if you travel a lot for work. One mother I have looked after was told she needed a yellow fever vaccination for travel for work – something that it is recommended you avoid during pregnancy – and her reluctance to have it was met with anger from her bosses. In this type of situation it is better to speak up and tell your employer that you are pregnant.

Another point that might be worth mentioning is that you may have close, trusted friends who you want to rely on if something does go wrong. I think it entirely appropriate to tell those friends.

coping with physical changes

High levels of hormones are the root cause of most of the signs of pregnancy (see page 24). You may get all the symptoms, a few, or none. All pregnancies are different. Below I go into more detail about the changes your body may experience, and offer some coping strategies and tips.

SORE OR ENLARGED BREASTS/TINGLING NIPPLES

First-time mothers especially might experience an extreme change in the size of their bust. Some mothers pregnant for a second or subsequent time say that they haven't seen as early or dramatic a change in their breast size, and some say they noticed barely any change at all in later pregnancies.

If you are struggling with enlarged and sore breasts, it's not too early to wear a maternity bra, which may feel much more comfortable and offer more support than a regular bra. Another tip is to wear a maternity bra to bed at night. Pregnant women are not supposed to wear under-wired bras.

You may grow several sizes before the end of your pregnancy and, as with maternity clothes, it's worth keeping in mind that you may not be this size for long before splashing out on new bras. I know many mothers who say their bra size went up 'one size every trimester, and then two sizes after the birth'.

A tingling sensation in the nipples is often cited as the first sign of pregnancy. However, a tingling sensation in one mother-to-be might be a sharp pain in the nipples of another. Other women find their nipples are very sensitive and sore in cold weather and that they need to put on extra vests or a wool jersey.

INCREASED VAGINAL DISCHARGE

This, again, can be a very early sign and is a universal symptom of pregnancy. The increase in thin, white and odourless discharge, or leucchorhea, is completely normal and caused by the increased turnover of the number of cells in the vaginal lining. A cause for concern is any discharge that causes discomfort, itching or burning, or that is foul-smelling or has any colour (greyish or greenish). See your GP for treatment.

As the body becomes more engorged, you may feel more interested in sex, experiencing heightened sensual awareness and more powerful orgasms. You may feel completely off sex, which is normal too.

IMPLANTATION BLEEDING (SPOTTING)

Not everyone experiences implantation bleeding, and some women have confused it for a period. Implantation bleeding is usually just a few spots of blood that is pink or brown in colour, and occurs about a week after you ovulate. It occurs as the fertilized egg embeds into the uterus, leading to a small amount of blood loss. It is not a cause for concern.

'Spotting' between six and eight weeks is also quite common and not always a cause for concern, but it is worth mentioning it to your doctor or midwife. Spotting accompanied by cramping and a loss of pregnancy symptoms should always be reported to your doctor.

METALLIC TASTE IN THE MOUTH

This is another first symptom for some. I know one mother, unexpectedly pregnant for the fourth time, who brushed her teeth furiously trying to get rid of the taste, before it dawned on her that she could be pregnant again.

AVERSION TO CERTAIN FOODS

In the same way that you can experience cravings, some women experience an extreme dislike of certain foods, which can continue after the pregnancy is over.

Many women have said they went off coffee or suddenly found it too strong tasting. Food aversions can be triggers for morning sickness. It's important to identify and avoid the triggers, especially if you are prone to vomiting. See the tips on coping with morning sickness on page 28.

SENSITIVITY TO STRONG SMELLS

Certain smells can produce a strong reaction. Ask those around you to be sensitive and not cook fatty foods, the most common trigger. Try to open a window or go outside to get a few gulps of fresh air. Cigarette smoke can also be a trigger. Avoid places where you might be exposed to smoke or ask people to smoke away from you.

EXCESS SALIVA (PTYALISM)

In some women this can be so pronounced that they are forced to carry a tissue with them to wipe away some of the excess. Keep plenty of tissues at hand if you want to spit it out discreetly. Like many of the symptoms of early pregnancy, it will pass.

TIREDNESS

Most women feel extraordinarily tired in the first trimester of pregnancy and it may be that you have never experienced anything like it. It is an overpowering exhaustion that can hit you like a brick wall, and it is usually more pronounced with subsequent pregnancies. Some women have compared it to jetlag, saying they felt their body was disorientated and out of sorts with its normal rhythm. Other women say it's similar to the feeling of being 'very hungover'. I describe it as an all-consuming exhaustion that hits you like the heat of a tropical climate when you step out of the plane. In the same way that being sick does not necessarily alleviate the nausea of morning sickness, sleep doesn't guarantee you'll wake up feeling refreshed. You may feel tired even after a fairly long rest.

Your body is working very hard and going through quite astronomical changes. There is the beginning of a new life inside you; blood is being pumped to support it, cell tissues are forming. Your body is rapidly adapting to these changes, and coping with a huge surge in hormones in your system. Progesterone is also said to have a sedative effect.

My advice is to gear your day around what you need to do, then rest. Catnaps can be grabbed at intervals if you are travelling by train or bus. Some offices have an Occupational Health Worker who may have an office you can rest in at lunchtime or late afternoon, depending on your hours.

If you are expected to do a lot of long-haul travel, you may need to tell your boss that you are in the first few weeks of pregnancy and get the travel cut back. Many women find it too much in the first trimester.

Another tip is to eat earlier in the evening so that you can go to bed earlier. If you work in an office, get home as soon as possible, take a relaxing bath, then get to bed as early as possible. Reorganize your social life so that you can cope: cut back on late nights – they will catch up with you.

If your partner likes to read, watch TV, talk on the phone or use the computer in the bedroom, you will have to ask them to adapt to the change in routine. I add here a plea to partners: tiredness is a huge issue, especially for a busy mother-to-be. A newly pregnant woman needs almost as much sleep as a child.

DIZZINESS AND FAINTING

I used to feel faint a lot when I was expecting and it is a very common symptom in women who have low blood pressure, which is often exacerbated by pregnancy. Dizziness and fainting can also go hand-in-hand with morning sickness. It's useful to employ a few coping rituals if you think you feel a faint coming on. The usual sign is sudden dizziness which, if left unchecked, will pass in front of the eyes like an out-of-tune television. You may feel a fuzzy sensation in your ears before the world goes black and you fall.

As soon as I felt a fainting spell coming on, I would go into my little ritual to prevent it. I would remove my shoes, get my feet onto a cold surface and/or wriggle my toes. I would then get my head down to a low level before I was at the point where I couldn't hear anymore. Usually this would stop me from actually passing out.

If you can't avoid the faint, try to warn someone so they can break your fall. If no one is around, try to fall to your knees to avoid falling on your bump. If you think you are going to faint while you are sitting down on a sofa, in the back of a car or on a bench, try lying down on your left side. If you are in a chair, try to slide forwards onto your knees. Another trick is to get into a doorway and hold the frame with both hands. You can then gently slide to your knees as you faint.

HEADACHES

Headaches are caused primarily by the huge hormonal changes in the body. Mostly, they will decrease after the first trimester, but for some they persist.

To avoid headaches, drink water regularly, eat small amounts often, and get plenty of fresh air. Try to avoid overheated environments, strong smells and long periods of standing up. If a headache is very bad, lie down in a darkened room, take some paracetamol and try to shut out the outside world. Gently massage your temples, the inner edges of your eyebrows and above your nose using gentle, circular motions.

If you work at a desk, remember to keep your feet flat on the floor and try to extend the space between your ears and your shoulders. To relieve tension, try rolling your shoulders, breathing slowly and deeply.

Aromatherapy oils that are recommended to relieve headaches include lavender, peppermint, ginger, rosemary and eucalyptus. For a homeopathic remedy, see your local practitioner. If headaches persist, see your GP, as you may need further investigations and treatment.

THE NEED TO PEE MORE OFTEN AND CONSTIPATION

The need to go to the loo more often is caused by pressure that is put on the bladder by your expanding uterus. It usually subsides at around 12 weeks, only

tips for relieving constipation

- ☉ Increase your fluid intake – drink plenty of water.
- ☉ Use linseeds – the trick here is to use one tablespoon of linseeds in two-thirds of a glass of water. The gunge that rises to the surface overnight can be put on top of food and greatly relieves constipation.
- ☉ Try eating bran (make sure you always complement bran with oily foods).
- ☉ Other foods that can help to relieve constipation are: prunes (including prune yoghurt), dried apricots (although too many can have the opposite effect), sweetcorn, mangoes, papaya, squash, beans, pulses and lentils, beetroot and Tabasco sauce.

to return later in pregnancy when the larger baby puts pressure on the bladder.

From around 14 weeks onwards you may feel constipated and, while this is essentially something for the second trimester, I want to put a warning about this here because it can lead to piles (haemorrhoids). Constipation can be aggravated in women who are prone to bowel irregularity or who have irritable bowel syndrome. The first point to remember is not to strain when you go to the loo. The second point is to watch your diet – you need a combination of roughage and oil to help lubricate the system. See the box, left, for some tips.

YOUR THICKENING TUMMY

At the end of the first trimester you may notice that you have lost your waist definition and that the whole area appears 'square'. The tummy is thickening and you may notice 'fat stores' around your hips, upper thighs, breasts and bottom. These fat stores are laid down in preparation for your milk production.

You may also have a bloated appearance, which is not yet quite a 'bump'. It's all very normal, very much part of pregnancy, and not forever. Tight clothing may make you feel worse so avoid it. Today there are plenty of things on the market that can help you adapt your clothes and feel comfortable in the first trimester without spending much money.

There is an elasticated 'button hook' which provides a bridge between button and hole when you are just a tiny bit too big for your jeans, but can't yet fit into maternity wear (see page 329 for sources). Jeans that are low slung can be worn for longer than those that are high waisted, and loose-fitting clothes are obviously more comfortable.

WEIGHT GAIN

Please don't diet. (See the information on eating disorders on page 65 if you are having trouble coping with weight gain.) Government advice is that most women should gain between 10kg and 12.5kg (22lb and 28lb) during pregnancy. That is often broken down as follows:

Weight of the baby	38 per cent
Weight of the placenta	9 per cent
Weight of the amniotic fluid	11 per cent
Increase in weight of the uterus and breasts	20 per cent
Increase in weight of the blood	22 per cent

In the first trimester the recommended weight gain is around 1.8kg (4lb), but I don't pay too much attention to the weight rules in the first trimester as it is a tricky time and it is impossible to have a 'one size fits all' rule. I've seen very skinny women put on far more than the amount recommended, but perhaps they needed to. Other women may find that they are losing weight in the first trimester because of sickness.

If you are of average weight then my own view is that you probably don't need to be weighed all the time in pregnancy, if at all. For normal women, a fixation with weight can be distracting and miss the point.

If you are underweight, my advice is that you may need to catch up – for you and your baby. If you are at the upper end of the scales, concentrate on growing your baby and limit your own drive to eat. Women who are either under- or overweight can have problems in pregnancy and birth. See the information on BMI on pages 64–5.

The important thing to remember is that you will get into your stride come the second trimester – that thickening around the tummy will turn into a lovely bump and you will soon feel 'pregnant' as opposed to just bloated.

CRAMPING

Some women describe a warm feeling in the lower abdomen and it is symptomatic of the amount of blood your body is pumping into the uterus. For some women this feeling can turn into a 'dragging sensation' when they have been doing too much. If you feel the mild cramping is getting worse the more you do, take some rest. You may well be overdoing it. Listen to your body.

If you have painful cramping, especially accompanied by spotting or bleeding, and a loss of pregnancy symptoms, tell your doctor immediately.

SEEMINGLY INSATIABLE HUNGER AND CRAZY CRAVINGS

Like the tiredness, the sudden hunger that takes over can be all consuming. While your body is swirling with hormones, you need to listen to it. Medical advice today is mixed. Some doctors argue that you don't need any extra calories for the first six months of pregnancy, and only the daily calorific equivalent of two extra slices of toast in the last three months (although some argue it is as much as 300 calories). The recommended daily amount of calories for women is 1,940, so it's a far cry from the 'eating for two' mentality of previous generations. That said, many women experience very strong hunger pangs in the first trimester, almost 'a drive to eat, and eat now'.

While the Department of Health have guidelines on healthy balanced eating, your body may have other ideas. I tend to go easy on women in the first trimester and push the 'sensible eating' patterns later, as this is a haphazard time. It may be that your body is craving pasta and mashed potatoes because carbohydrates are what you need right now.

It's quite normal to adopt some strange eating habits in the early stages of pregnancy; my own craving was for Tabasco sauce, which I shook liberally on everything. Some women find themselves craving foods that they wouldn't normally touch, such as crisps saturated in artificial colouring, tinned exotic fruits and even ice. Others are good at translating their cravings into healthy food: ice cream equals a need for calcium, so perhaps try pasteurized cheese or a mug of hot milk sweetened with honey. A craving for crisps might be sated with cracker bread or Ryvita; black chocolate may mean your body is demanding iron, so try well-washed spinach or watercress salad.

If you are craving a lot of sugar in the form of chocolate, cakes and biscuits it could be your body's way of coping with the extraordinary tiredness. It's worth noting that sugar can make matters worse and put you into a cycle of a sugar high followed by a crash, which can result in you putting on unnecessary amounts of weight. If you are constantly craving sugar, try nuts and dried fruit, which will also fill you up. Perhaps introduce slow-burn carbohydrates to your diet, such as oats (found in some cereals, porridge and oat cakes) or lentils.

Fundamentally, you need to have a healthy eating plan in place by 16 weeks as this is when the hCG hormone goes down and the crazier cravings subside. The

pregnancy hormones

In pregnancy, the cocktail of hormones is quite potent. They have both physical and emotional side effects, and some women feel as if they have been literally robbed of their personalities as a result of all this biological activity. At other times in pregnancy, it is the hormones that can make us feel blissfully happy and content. They provide those tidal waves of love that come crashing over us in the early weeks after birth, when exhaustion would otherwise have got the better of us.

HCG (HUMAN CHORIONIC GONADOTROPIN) This is the hormone that pregnancy tests detect and it is vital in early pregnancy. Shortly after conception it is produced by the embryo, and later by a part of the placenta. Its role is to maintain progesterone production and some scientists believe that it stops the body's immune system from rejecting the embryo.

PROGESTERONE Progesterone is essential for, among other things, maintaining the function of the placenta. It also helps drive the mood swings and is partly responsible for tiredness as it can have a sedative effect. It is, in conjunction with a group of hormones called oestrogen, one of the most important hormones for women generally and in pregnancy. Progesterone and oestrogen levels build as pregnancy progresses and, along with relaxin, they have a profound effect on muscles, ligaments and joints, helping them to relax and loosen in preparation for your growing bump and for the birth.

OESTROGEN is responsible for making your breasts grow, and for maturing the baby's lungs, kidneys, liver, adrenal gland and other organs. It also promotes blood flow through the uterus. A positive side effect of oestrogen is the 'pregnancy glow', caused by an increase in blood volume to the vessels beneath the skin.

RELAXIN This group of hormones allows your vaginal and pelvic floor muscles to stretch.

OXYTOCIN 'The love hormone' is released in response to touching and orgasm in both men and women. In labour, oxytocin causes the uterus to contract. Oxytocin is also central to the 'let down' reflex during breastfeeding.

PROLACTIN This hormone has many roles. After birth, when progesterone levels in your body drop, prolactin allows milk to flow to the breast.

ENDORPHINS These are released during exercise and when you are happy and help you feel positive. In labour they act as natural pain relief.

placenta takes over and you'll feel more in control of your diet. See the section on changing your diet, pages 30–1.

MOOD SWINGS, INCLUDING 'TEARS FOR NO REASON'

Hormones, hormones! It's easy to feel that the hormones have taken control (and in many respects, they have). Your body is coping, in some cases, with a hundred times the normal amount of hormones in its system (see opposite). This can produce an extraordinary range of feelings: Zen-like calmness; heart-bursting elation; heightened sensitivity; raging fury; stubborn indignation; unexplained sadness; even mild depression. You may also be prone to bouts of inexplicable crying, become oversensitive or feel injustices keenly. Some women have described their urge to say everything that comes into their head as 'pregnancy Tourette's', referring to the syndrome that causes sufferers to exclaim either obscene or socially inappropriate remarks.

It is not uncommon to shy away from watching 'bad stories' on the news or being super-sensitive to issues concerning children. Another common feeling is sudden anger, quickly followed by a spell of tears and a helpless feeling summarized by the phrase 'but I'm pregnant!'. This is all normal.

Like most of the symptoms of pregnancy, there are ways of coping with the mood swings. You need to take a step back from the situation and remember those hormones rushing through your body. If you fear the hormones may influence a serious decision at work, a social situation or influence your urge to say something that may be insensitive, put it off until you have had time to reflect or sleep on it. The situation may look entirely different in the morning.

Try taking a deep breath and restoring calm within. This is a very good time to practise some visualisation techniques (see pages 71–3, 128 and 168).

Let patience wash over you and keep taking deep breaths. Think to yourself that this is good practice for motherhood. The ability to stay calm will be particularly useful when you are exhausted and trying to work out why the baby is crying. Even when you feel totally helpless, it's important to take deep breaths and take control of the situation again.

MISGIVINGS ABOUT THE PREGNANCY

I have included a section on this under moodswings because such misgivings can result in the mother becoming quite depressed. While a pregnancy, particularly one that has been worked at, is an occasion for great joy, it is not always as simple as that. Many of us have spent time in our lives trying not to get pregnant. You may also have gone through a period of wondering if 'now' was the right time. You may have then thought you would like to be pregnant and, when it doesn't happen immediately, wondered 'will I ever be?'

Pregnancy is a complicated issue in modern society. Consequently, some women are overwhelmed by misgivings. They feel they can't talk about this ambivalence because it is 'not done' to feel regret about a wanted pregnancy (especially if you have friends who are undergoing fertility treatment). Nonetheless, you may feel 'what have I done?'

Your emotional response to your pregnancy may take you completely by surprise – I've had many women who have said, 'I don't know if I want to be pregnant and yet we'd been trying for a baby for such a long time.' Many women feel anxious too, about how their body will change, about the baby's welfare, about the birth and how they will cope after the birth, both financially and emotionally. Approach these feelings one at a time and try to get some perspective. Talk to your partner or a good friend – perhaps someone who has been through it?

When the pregnancy is unplanned it may feel like too much of a shock. It's helpful to remember that sometimes – often, even – babies come at unplanned or unpredictable times.

If you are in a complicated situation and your thoughts are in a muddle, you need to start by unravelling the situation and looking at it bit by bit. Take a step back. Perhaps you have recently lost your job; perhaps you are a student in the middle of a course. You are not alone. Women everywhere are making decisions about how this tiny baby will fit into their lives. Every day, women face these situations and cope. While it is an enormous responsibility to bring a child into the world, it is entirely manageable – women have been doing it for millennia. Try to think positively: you can overcome obstacles. These things happen all the time and it does get sorted out. You will find your own way. Confide in someone experienced to help you get some perspective. Talk to your GP and perhaps ask to be referred for counselling.

One of the first hurdles is acceptance. The journey of pregnancy and the act of bringing a baby into the world is one of the most unpredictable times of life. It is a potent cocktail and it will probably give you the best as well as the toughest times of life. Certainly my own experience was that my first baby was at once the most difficult and the most wonderful thing.

MORNING SICKNESS

It is the most widely recognized, the most widely researched and, most women would agree, perhaps the most debilitating of what are professionally termed 'the minor disorders of pregnancy'.

Morning sickness is thought to affect anywhere between 50% and 85% of pregnant women from six weeks' gestation. It can range from faint nausea at any time of day to regular and severe vomiting. Only 0.5% of women suffer from hyperemesis gravidarum, which is an extreme form of morning sickness that requires hospital treatment to avoid dehydration.

It may come as little comfort, but old wisdom has it that a queasy pregnancy is a good pregnancy. This has been backed up by medical research that shows women with morning sickness have a reduced risk of miscarriage and are more likely to have a healthy baby (although of course it does not automatically follow that the absence of morning sickness equals a bad pregnancy).

As we all know, morning sickness is a misnomer. It can attack at anytime of day. It is also not a 'sickness', but a thoroughly normal symptom of pregnancy. Medical research has mixed views on its causes, but research by scientists at Cornell University in New York[1] suggests that morning sickness is nature's way of protecting the mother from food that may be dangerous to the growing foetus while its major organ systems are developing in the first trimester. While a pregnant woman's immune system is down (in order to prevent her rejecting the baby as a foreign tissue), the nausea and aversions protect her from toxins that may be more prevalent in some foods.

Interestingly, many women feel 'off' meat, fish and eggs in the first three months which, as well as being good sources of protein, can also carry risks if they are not properly prepared or stored. The biologists at Cornell found that the percentage of women suffering from morning sickness was higher in Japan where the staple diet, raw fish, can be harmful to a developing foetus.

Coffee, too, has been found, in high doses, to increase the risk of miscarriage and, perhaps unsurprisingly, it is one of the most common food aversions cited by pregnant women. Similarly, studies have shown that few pregnant women crave alcohol, which can cause Foetal Alcohol Syndrome. Most women agree that very bland foods, such as cereals and bread, are easiest to stomach. I have also seen extreme cases where women can only eat baby food.

So, despite the fact that you feel awful, it may be helpful to remember that this is your body working naturally to protect your baby. It is a magical time and it is important to try to be positive. In the vast majority of cases the nausea subsides by 12 weeks and, believe it or not, by 16 weeks some women struggle to remember how bad it was.

Note for second or third timers: all pregnancies are different. Some women are nausea-free for their first and sick as a dog with their second, regardless of the baby's sex. Morning sickness can also be genetic and, if your mother was a sufferer, you may be more likely to have it.

combating queasiness

There are many practical ways to combat queasiness, depending on the severity. Here are some that I have seen work:

- ⊙ drink water: fizzy water might prove more effective
- ⊙ sleep: tiredness can exacerbate morning sickness
- ⊙ keep digestive biscuits, oatcakes or crackers by the bed to eat before you get out of bed. This helps counteract acid and is also good for blood sugar
- ⊙ try ginger tea, ginger beer and/or ginger biscuits – ginger has recognized anti-sickness properties
- ⊙ as with ginger, peppermint is said to relieve nausea – try a couple of drops of peppermint oil on a hankie, peppermint tea or sucking peppermint sweets
- ⊙ some women swear by lemons – add a slice of lemon to your tea
- ⊙ eat small meals frequently – hunger, oddly enough, can actually be a trigger for morning sickness and eating, even when food is the last thing you feel like, can be a great help
- ⊙ stick to bland, non-fatty foods that won't upset your system; avoid anything rich, spicy or too acidic
- ⊙ if you smoke, give up now. It can make morning sickness worse
- ⊙ try an acupressure wristband, available from most chemists – a small button presses on the pressure point that is said to relieve nausea. Some of the women I've looked after wear one on each wrist and then fiddle with them as a form of distraction from the sickness, too.

ACNE

Acne is a common symptom of early pregnancy and is caused, as it is in teenage years, by hormones that make your skin produce more oil. If you are taking fertility drugs such as Clomid the acne may be worse.

Take solace in the fact that this is usually only a symptom of the first trimester, and in a couple of months the acne will have given way to the wonderful pregnancy 'glow' you've heard about.

You must be careful with what you use to treat acne – many products are contraindicated with pregnancy. If you are taking prescribed drugs to treat acne when you discover you are pregnant, speak to your GP immediately. Drugs such as Roaccutane and Oxytetracycline must not be taken during pregnancy.

Some women find that their acne clears up during pregnancy.

PREGNANCY AMNESIA

You may find that you are suddenly very scatty and can't concentrate properly or remember things, such as people's names, dates, appointments or even which day of the week it is. This can be frustrating for very organized women, but it's nothing to be concerned about. It's a perfectly normal symptom of pregnancy caused by increasing levels of endorphins in your system.

My advice is to write everything down. Check your diary regularly and keep lists. If there is something very important that you are worried you may forget, use Post-it notes somewhere you will see them, such as on the fridge.

changing your diet

Like so many areas of pregnancy and birth, the list of what you can and can't eat is always the subject of debate. While the advice seems to greatly differ depending on your country of origin, culture and beliefs, there is one certainty – that a healthy, balanced diet is obviously the best diet. And make sure you take folic acid supplements. Folic acid supplements have been shown to reduce incidence of babies being born with spina bifida, a defect of the spinal cord.

When eating out, be careful in restaurants or cafes where you have not seen the food prepared. Use common sense. Don't eat anywhere that looks filthy or where you feel uncomfortable. And don't rely on waiting staff to know what is on or off the menu for pregnant women.

foods to avoid

Some foods can be dangerous during pregnancy and should be avoided. Below I give a list of these foods as per the UK government guidelines.

RAW AND UNDERCOOKED EGGS
These are off the menu because of the risk of salmonella food poisoning. Raw eggs are found in home-made mayonnaise, ice cream, cheesecake and mousse-type puddings.

UNPASTEURIZED MILK OR CHEESE AND BLUE CHEESE
The advice on pasteurized cheese differs depending where you live. However, the risk of listeria is particularly dangerous to an unborn child, so it's better to avoid these foods. Even a mild form of the illness can cause miscarriage, stillbirth or severe illness in the newborn.

PÂTÉ
Even vegetable pâté is off the menu. Foie gras (goose liver pâté) and meat terrines are also forms of pâté. These foods carry a risk of listeria (see above). Also, foie gras is very high in Vitamin A, which can be harmful to your baby.

toxoplasmosis

It's not only certain foods that carry a risk of toxoplasmosis. You also need to be cautious with cat and dog poo and when gardening. If you have a pet, use rubber gloves to deal with their faeces. The same applies when gardening; wear gloves to avoid contracting toxoplasmosis.

LIVER OR LIVER PRODUCTS

This includes liver pâté and liver sausage. The government recommends you avoid this because of high levels of Vitamin A that could be harmful to your baby.

RAW AND UNDERCOOKED MEAT

Obviously undercooked poultry is something you would always avoid, but it is particularly important during pregnancy because of the risk of toxoplasmosis (caused by a parasite called toxoplasma gondii, which can be found in raw meat), which can harm your baby. Make sure there are no traces of 'pink' or blood in the chicken you cook or eat, and hot wash all surfaces and utensils after preparing raw meat. Lamb and beef should be served well-done and not pink or rare.

SHARK, MARLIN AND SWORDFISH, AND RAW FISH (SUSHI)

These fish contain mercury in high levels that could interrupt your baby's developing nervous system.

TUNA AND 'OILY' FISH

Tuna should be limited to one serving per week because of the high mercury count. Oily fish, such as salmon, mackerel, sardines and trout, should be limited to two servings per week.

RAW SHELLFISH

Be cautious with cooked shellfish (e.g. mussels, cockles, clams, crab, prawns and scallops to name a few) and avoid raw shellfish altogether as it can contain harmful bacteria and viruses that could cause food poisoning.

UNWASHED FRUIT, VEGETABLES AND SALADS

You need to wash fruit, vegetables and salad thoroughly to get rid of all soil as it may contain toxoplasma and lead to toxoplasmosis (see above).

changing your lifestyle

Attitudes that you adopt to keep you and your baby healthy in pregnancy can help you to change bad habits for good. They will improve your health in the long run, and set a good example for your child in the years to come.

DIET

Now that you are starting a family it's a good time to examine your basic eating habits. When there was only one or two of you, it may have been easy to pick up a microwave meal on the way home from work. Family meals, however, require more planning and you may as well start this approach now. After all, you want to put good, healthy food into your children's pure systems. You can start with simple modifications and get more adventurous as you gain confidence. If you can't cook, perhaps now is the time to start trying – healthy, home-made food is better in the end for your children.

EXERCISE

Even if you can't face it between feeling sick and overwhelming tiredness, I do believe it's important to introduce some exercise, preferably very gentle exercise if you are not used to it. Don't use pregnancy as an excuse for sitting on your bottom; your body needs to be in shape. Equally don't do anything too strenuous and exhaust yourself. Even walking that extra stop on the bus route can make a difference. If you are stuck in a stuffy room looking at a VDU all day, get out and have a walk in the fresh air. Walking can be wonderful for your lower back and pelvis and many pregnant women feel it really helps them unwind, especially in later weeks.

Swimming is helpful and also relaxing. What about a gentle swim in the local pool when you feel up to it?

The first trimester is a great time to find out where there are classes locally for pregnancy yoga or pregnancy Pilates. Many classes don't allow women to start until after 20 weeks but they may book up early so it's worth finding out and getting your place booked.

Remember – labour is like running a marathon and it's good to get preparation in early. Exercise can also be helpful in making 'the head stronger than the uterus' (see pages 71–3).

lifestyle for pregnancy; lifestyle for life

Perhaps you and your partner are smokers or drink over the recommended weekly limit of alcohol. Perhaps you like staying up late at night; you may, occasionally, dabble in recreational drugs. If any of these things apply to you, you need to take a long look at your life. None of these bad habits sit well with the arrival of a tiny baby. Nor does it help if one of you changes your life but the other remains stuck in the old ways. It's good to start acting as a team now – after all, teamwork is essential for good parenting.

Sit down together and work out how you can change patterns that may have developed into bad habits. Start by gently changing your weekly habits – instead of the pub on a Friday evening that may end up in a late night 'session' why not go to the cinema? Weekend walks can be a great time for bonding and for planning for the future. How about one of you cooks a meal for the other one day a week? New patterns need not be boring to be good for you. Work out ways to have fun in a healthy way and these new ideas will become new habits quickly and easily.

As for letting go of the old ways, see the information below on smoking and drinking, and the information on preparing for parenthood (see pages 39–48) for advice.

SMOKING

Evidence on smoking in pregnancy is clear – it will harm your baby. If you smoke while pregnant you are at higher risk of having a stillbirth or a premature or underweight baby that is at higher risk of infection and even cot death.

When you smoke a cigarette a cocktail of poisons is passed to your baby, including carbon monoxide. Your baby will have trouble getting oxygen and, in effect, be coughing and spluttering. The nicotine will also speed up his or her heart rate. Babies born to smoking mothers are more likely to suffer from asthma, chest infections, coughs and colds and are more likely to be smokers themselves in later life.

The sooner you stop, the better. Ask your partner, family and friends for support. If anyone else in your house smokes, ask them to smoke outside, or, better still, to give up too. A house full of cigarette smoke is no place for a newborn baby. (See page 327 for sources of support for quitting.)

DRINKING

Heavy or frequent drinking can seriously harm your baby. Alcohol is passed to the baby through the placenta, but the baby is not equipped to process it. Too much alcohol can cause Foetal Alcohol Syndrome – which means your baby may have restricted growth, facial deformity, heart defects, learning disabilities and behavioural problems. The current government advice was updated in August 2008 to advise no drinking at all during pregnancy.

My own advice has always been to avoid spirits completely, but that a small amount of wine or beer occasionally is fine. You should not drink more than two units (small glasses of wine) more than once or twice a week, and you should not get drunk. Again, ask for support from your partner, family or friends and don't ever let anyone pressurize you into having a drink.

If you have enjoyed a particularly boozy lifestyle up until now, it's time to revise it. After all, once you have a small baby to look after, a trip to the pub may not be your priority. If you are having trouble cutting down, see page 327 for sources of support.

DRUGS

Do not take any drugs during pregnancy, no matter how small the amount. All drugs, including cannabis, cross the placenta and can harm your baby. It is very important to tell your midwife or medical practitioner if you are addicted to drugs and to get immediate help. (See page 327 for sources of support.)

STAYING PURE

It may be obvious to you that the chemicals in household cleaning products, paints and varnishes etc, should be treated with caution when you are pregnant. However, it is not just the obvious that we need to treat with care.

In the age we live in, chemicals, such as those in hair dyes, nail varnish, fake tan and skin products, are difficult to avoid. Even some 'natural' products, such as oils and creams made from Tea Tree, and aromatherapy oils, may not be recommended in pregnancy.

Before you continue with your usual beauty routine, if you have one, make sure you tell your hairdresser, beautician, dermatologist or masseuse that you are pregnant. Highlighting your hair may be acceptable, for example, but strong bleaches next to the scalp, are not – in case the chemicals get into the blood stream. For this reason too, spray tans should be avoided. Unfortunately for those who like a constant tan, sunbeds are also out of the question – not just because skin reacts differently when you are pregnant but also because early reports into the effects of strong UV light suggests that it may deplete levels of folic acid in your system, which is not good for the developing embryo/foetus.

Botox injections are an absolute no-no, as are some skin preparations and creams. Try the 'stay pure' approach and, if your beauty professional doesn't know the answer, err on the side of caution.

your attitude to weight gain

I see a lot of women who are very concerned about the idea of putting on weight during pregnancy. I feel it's important to address these concerns here, as well as more serious problems such as eating disorders.

Perhaps the reason why this is such a concern is a sad off-shoot of a culture that is obsessed with appearance and weight, particularly when it comes to pregnant women. Perhaps there is a competitive element – a feeling that, 'my friend was thin while she was pregnant, I want to be thin too.' These fears and thoughts can colour some women's whole view of pregnancy. Every woman is different and every woman will 'carry' her baby differently. In a healthy pregnancy there is no good or bad. Enjoy your own pregnancy and love the changes in your own body that is nurturing your baby.

Worrying about your weight can also hugely exacerbate pregnancy symptoms – if you don't eat properly you may feel morning sickness more acutely, you may feel more exhausted and you may be more prone to fainting and dizziness.

It's important to remember that a pregnant woman is not fat, but pregnant. It is a positive, wonderful experience. Try to concentrate on what is happening inside, not outside. Visualize the little life growing inside you (see pages 49–52) and the idea that your baby will soon be kicking and gurgling in your arms. As your bump grows, stroke it and love it. It's your baby and it's part of you. You are growing it and looking after it. Let go of any negative thoughts you may be having about your changing body. (See page 327 for sources of help for people with eating disorders.)

medication

My view has always been that, during pregnancy, you should avoid medicines and opt for the natural approach where possible. It's best to play safe and treat all medicines as dangerous until you have consulted a doctor or pharmacist. Many medicines are not recommended for use in pregnancy including cough mixtures, antacids and cold remedies that you can buy over the counter.

That said, you should not allow a fever to go untreated. A fever can be dangerous to a foetus and can contribute to miscarriage. Take paracetamol (see below) to bring down a fever. You can also use old-fashioned remedies such as sponging your brow with tepid water and sleeping with minimal clothing and sheets. If it continues for more than 24 hours, see a doctor.

PAIN RELIEF

Paracetamol is considered safe in pregnancy, but no more than two at a time and eight in one day with four-hourly gaps. Most drugs, including asprin and Ibuprofen (Nurofen) are not to be taken during pregnancy.

ANTIBIOTICS AND OTHER MEDICATIONS

If you need to take antibiotics, ensure the doctor knows that you are pregnant.

If you are on prescribed medicine for a serious condition or illness, such as epilepsy, diabetes or bi-polar disorder, do not stop your medication, but see your doctor or specialist as soon as possible.

COMPLEMENTARY MEDICINE

It is not an automatic 'given' that all natural remedies are safe in pregnancy. If you are using aromatherapy or herbal or homeopathic medicine, ensure you tell your qualified practitioner that you are pregnant.

VACCINATIONS

Most medical professionals advise against vaccinations during pregnancy. If it is essential for you to travel to a country where vaccinations are required, speak to your GP. In some cases the risk of disease outweighs that of taking the vaccine. Vaccinations that are unsafe during pregnancy include yellow fever, polio, typhoid (when administered orally) and MMR (measles, mumps and rubella).

preparing your body for birth

Keeping fit during pregnancy will help you maintain good health and physical comfort as your body grows, and can also improve your birth experience by keeping you strong and fit enough to deal with it physically.

ADJUSTING YOUR EXERCISE ROUTINE

The type of exercise that is best for you during pregnancy depends on your level of fitness and your own inclinations. Avoid any exercise during which you can fall or sustain a 'bump to your bump', such as horse riding, skiing or kickboxing.

If you have an existing exercise regime that is rigorous, you will need to tone it down to a safe level. Talk to your fitness instructor or GP for advice.

STARTING AN EXERCISE ROUTINE

If you don't exercise, this is a good time to start. Begin with gentle exersion and build up slowly. Perhaps walk for an hour each day, building up speed over time.

YOUR PELVIC FLOOR

The pelvic floor is the sling of membrane and muscles that support your uterus and your bowel (see diagram on page 38). During pregnancy it needs to support the considerable weight of your growing uterus, and the pelvic floor takes quite a battering during vaginal delivery, and there is now evidence to show that your pelvic floor is damaged even if you have a Caesarean section.

Pelvic floor exercises are, therefore, essential during pregnancy. They should be practised whenever and wherever possible. I recommend you find a memory trigger to remind you to practise them. If you drive a lot, use a red traffic light. You can do them after a trip to the loo (make sure you have completely finished as it is not recommended to stop peeing mid-flow), when the phone rings or whenever you have a cup of tea. Turn it into a little ritual to help you remember. While it's true that you can 'overdo' pelvic floor exercises, it is pretty difficult.

FINDING YOUR PELVIC FLOOR There are two areas to think about, the 'front passage' and the 'back passage'. To find the front area, try to imagine you are stopping a pee mid-flow (although don't actually do this). Pull up and squeeze that area as if it were a sponge, and then hold for the count of three.

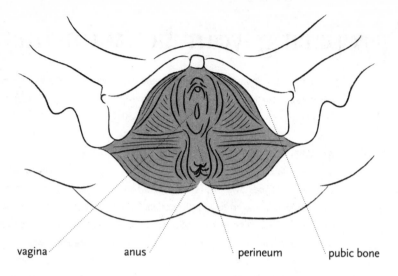

vagina   anus   perineum   pubic bone

Try to do this 10 times, breathing out slowly as you squeeze. To find the back area, imagine you are holding in wind. This area is sometimes easier to locate and it feels like a circle as opposed to the oval shape of the front area. Again pull up and squeeze for the count of three and then release. Then move into the middle for vaginal muscles. These are more difficult to locate, and are best identified during penetrative sex when you tighten them. Once you clearly recognize them, practise pulling them up and squeezing as you do for the pelvic floor muscles.

You can then do 10 quick squeezes of each. I call this a 'set' of exercises, and you want to aim for three sets in a day, if possible, although anything you can manage is a bonus. The first time you attempt a pelvic floor exercise you may find yourself clenching your jaw muscles, making a fist or tensing your legs at the same time. You need to relax your whole body and focus only on the area in question.

Pelvic floor exercises are the kind of thing you find embarrassing before pregnancy, but fully appreciate afterwards. Anyway, no one else will be able to tell when you are practising them.

preparing for parenthood

The beginning of pregnancy is a good time to consider the 'theory' of becoming a parent as part of preparation for parenthood as, later in pregnancy, practical considerations will be more pressing.

becoming a mother

'I am going to be a mother' – what does that mean? There must be a million definitions for what it means to become a mother. I heard a woman describe holding her baby for the first time as 'hugging a vast universe'. Another said it meant 'that I can never watch or hear the news in the same way again'. Her baby was born shortly before the tsunami on Boxing Day 2004 and she had spent three weeks in tears over the extraordinary loss of life – particularly of babies and children. I recently met a new mother who was bemused that she suddenly cared far less about her own wardrobe and appearance, and more about the future of the planet, 'which I hadn't given a second thought to before'. A mother who held strong political beliefs, said: 'It's funny how all your principles go out of the window once you have children. I was strongly in favour of state schools. Now I have a child, I'm considering the possibility of private education, which I never thought I would do.'

Becoming a mother often means developing a heightened sensitivity to the feelings of children, which can be traumatic and cause great anxiety, but is also part of what makes that 'mothering instinct'. These 'instincts' are in part biological, caused by natural hormonal changes in our systems that prepare us for motherhood and then help us through the early weeks. As well as boundless, almost suffocating love, they promote the desire to nurture, to protect ferociously, to empathize and to feel positive about life.

There are a huge range of other complex emotions involved in the 'mothering instinct' – a sense of responsibility, huge pride, a feeling of maturity, of being 'bound to the world', perhaps even a sharpened awareness of your own upbringing. Some women said they felt 'softer' after having children, and 'more forgiving' of the world around them. Others feel closer to their mothers – or, in some instances, hurt and upset by their mothers. A few have strongly negative feelings towards anyone they feel has caused hurt to children. The arrival of this tiny thing will certainly mean you recalibrate your priorities in life, and some things may come as a surprise – expect the unexpected.

becoming a father

Becoming a Dad can, dare I say it, bring about an even wider range of emotions than becoming a mum. Dads-to-be, it's a good idea to get to grips with these emotions and concerns now, so that you can be as prepared and involved as possible during the coming months.

Men often say that their first emotion is quite basic – the 'whoah, look how virile I am' response, quickly followed by joy/shock/fear, usually all rolled into one. Some men say they suffer 'sympathy symptoms' – tiredness, irritability, a huge increase in appetite and even backache. This is normal. Other men feel confused and slightly alienated by the whole process. They wonder, 'what is my role now? I'm not pregnant and the baby won't be here for ages.' They may feel their 'partner in crime' has gone – who will they share an evening drink with now? They may feel lost, or even bored if their partner suddenly falls asleep at 9 o'clock. They may feel their pregnant partner is irrational and too emotional – that sense of 'everything I say is wrong and she won't stop crying'.

Pregnancy can be a highly complicated and emotional journey for both Mum and Dad, but there is one crucial thing to remember: teamwork. Good parenting is all about working together. My advice on what you can do now is, support each other. 'Being supportive' takes many shapes. While your partner is looking after the baby inside her, you can look after her. If you live together, you can get her something to eat and drink in the morning, help her if she's feeling sick, make sure supper is planned when she gets back from work. You can patiently listen to her complaints, get a video for you both, run her a bath, even provide her with a gentle massage – if she wants one (some women hate to be touched during pregnancy).

When you are alone together, think of conversations that bring you both together – thoughts about the birth, names for the baby, plans for the future and so on. You may be moving house. If so, can you share the load when it comes to organizing, decorating, choosing new furniture, etc? What else can you do to relieve some of her workload?

It's true that many men complain that they have to put up with being a verbal punch bag when she is ratty and tired in the first trimester. Remember – this phase is short-lived, and hormonal rages are best met with patience, kindness, good humour and understanding (even when you want to just leave the house).

PATERNAL RESPONSIBILITY

A more long-term issue for many men is the idea of responsibility. The burden, particularly of financial responsibility, can be overwhelming, as can be the pressure to be a good 'role model'. Men, as well as women, often have to 'declutter' their lives in advance of the new arrival. It may be that you need to think carefully about finances, even question your current job if it's not enough to cover living costs for a small family. The sooner this is addressed, the stronger your position will be, and the more relaxed and in control you will feel about the baby's arrival.

Another unexpected emotion I have heard men express is about their sense of 'self-worth'. Some men suddenly question their own abilities, knowledge of the world and of life in general, when they picture their son or daughter looking up at them for guidance. One man told me, 'When my wife told me she was pregnant, one of my first emotions was a bizarre fear that I would have a son who wanted to play football with me in the park. I am rubbish at football – I'm rubbish at all sports. I was afraid that I would fail him, that I couldn't live up to the expectations of being "a Dad". Once he was born, I quickly got over not fulfilling this stereotype and realized there are so many other things I have to offer. I changed his nappy more than my wife in the first few weeks. Being a Dad, thank God, is about so much more than football.'

Fathers Direct (see page 328 for contact details) offers support to fathers.

single motherhood

There are many reasons why you may find yourself alone and bringing up a child or children. Fortunately, society is far more open-minded about single mothers today. They are generally recognized as a vulnerable group who need protection and support from outside. If you are single and pregnant, you may need to turn to family and friends for support – and my advice is, don't be shy.

Don't try to be brave. You and your baby need support, and you deserve it.

Even if you are secure financially, you need to think about emotional support. You may have issues to resolve in relation to the father. You may feel abandoned; you may not want him to play a role. Obviously it would be better to resolve whatever issues you can before the baby is born. This may even involve making your peace with the situation alone – you can ask your doctor to refer you for counselling to help you cope.

Some women choose to go it alone, and even set out to conceive without a partner, either through fertility treatment or through a casual encounter. Regardless of how single-minded you felt when you set out to get pregnant, you will probably find you need support as the pregnancy wears on. If you cannot turn to family or friends, try to organize a one-to-one midwife. Express your concerns and fears about being a single mother at your hospital booking or community appointment.

I can offer a word of reassurance: I have looked after many single mothers, in many different situations and the vast majority found a way of coping throughout the pregnancy and, often beautifully, during the birth.

The organization Gingerbread (see page 328 for contact details) may be useful.

teenage mums

This country has the highest rate of 'teenage pregnancies' (babies born to women aged under 18[2]) in Europe, at between 42–48 births per 1,000. Research also shows that if your mother was a teenage mum, you have a slightly increased chance of having your first child in your teens.

My first piece of advice is this – tell someone immediately if you think you are pregnant. Medically speaking, teenage mums are a vulnerable 'high risk' group and need to be seen at the hospital as soon as possible. They need proper help and care. Their own bodies are still immature and they are at a higher risk of pre-eclampsia. Many teenage mums try to conceal their pregnancies and that factor can bring its own complications. It's important that these young women feel safe and cared for, and that they get the help they need as soon as possible.

It is also essential that all aspects of caring for a newborn are explained to and understood by a teenage mother.

If you are a teenage mum, make sure you are as informed as possible about your situation. Ask questions and then ask more questions. Midwives will offer support and will schedule your pregnancy appointments and antenatal classes to meet your needs. Support is also available if you need help to stop smoking, taking drugs or drinking alcohol. You can continue to go to school and will not be excluded because of the pregnancy. If you wish to continue at school after the baby arrives, financial support is available to pay for childcare costs.

Who's the father? There will also be ramifications here, particularly if he is a teenage father. How will he provide financial support? Will his parents be involved? The behaviour of the father can also be very hard on a teenage mum, and you will need support and advice on how to cope with it.

See page 328 for organizations that may be useful. And speak to your hospital about how to get in touch with other teenage and young mums.

CASE STUDY **TEENAGE MUM**

'I had always thought teenage mums were stupid. We all know how not to get pregnant. I would've probably looked down at anyone at school who was pregnant. Then I left school at 15 – with one GCSE that I'd taken early – and I met my boyfriend. I'd only known my boyfriend for three months and we were using a very laid-back form of contraception, but it was still a shock.

There was no question in my mind that I would keep it. I didn't try and hide my pregnancy. My parents were shocked but supportive. My dad came with me to a lot of the antenatal appointments.

I was 16 but I looked a lot younger so people really stared at me. I would hear the disapproving comments and people would deliberately not get up for me on the bus. They would be very rude. They would ask me how old I was and if I knew the father. Maybe because of the stigma I felt I had to go out of the way to show how responsible I was. I was really strict with the diet, I wouldn't eat mushrooms in case they were dirty, and I didn't touch a drop of alcohol, even on my birthday. I went to all my appointments and to the classes, and my boyfriend came too. I remember them saying that when you first have signs of labour to carry on as normal and do the shopping and make something to eat.

I had contractions on and off for a couple of weeks and then the day my boyfriend and I moved in together I went into labour. The hospital was quite a long way and I kept saying that we had to go, but he'd taken the antenatal classes to heart and really wanted me to go to the supermarket. Finally I got to hospital and they asked me how long I'd been in labour. When I told them they looked disappointed and said I might have to go home and that I could be in for a long wait.

Then a midwife came to check me and I was 9cm. The labour was six and a half hours in total, quite short. I stuck to my plan and went in the pool for a bit and had some gas and air. I'd brought oils and a burner and that was nice. The thing I didn't like was that all these people kept "popping in" to look at me.

When I was a "new mum" people were even more direct with their questions – when I went out people would ask if the baby was my sister and then be really shocked when I said she was my daughter.

I felt lonely because I'd moved out of home to live with my boyfriend, but he had to work all hours to afford to keep us so I spent loads of time on my own with a new baby. I didn't see anyone. In the end my boyfriend and I started fighting – I think we both realized it wasn't working. I moved back in with my mum after eight months.

When my daughter was old enough I took her to a childminder while I did an Access course and then a degree. I decided I had to finish my education because otherwise I wouldn't be able to argue that she had to stay and finish school. She's now at school and I'm working. It hasn't been easy but I've turned it around and I'm proud of what I've achieved.' AMY, 22

> 'When my daughter was old enough ... I decided I had to finish my education because otherwise I wouldn't be able to argue that she had to stay and finish school. She's now at school and I'm working. It hasn't been easy but I'm proud of what I've achieved.'

financial responsibilities

Many couples have to make considerable sacrifices in their spending and reorganize their finances to make room for the enormous cost of having a baby. Ask yourself how you will cope with the financial responsibilities a baby brings. Besides the things you need to have ready for a newborn baby (see pages 108–9), you may also be thinking ahead to costs such as the endless supplies of nappies, wipes, toiletries, clothes etc, and the cost of childcare when and if you go back to work.

Try making an honest list of all your outgoings and see what is left over. You may need to sacrifice a few nights out, your clothes allowance or plans to redecorate the kitchen. There are hundreds of ways to save money if you apply your imagination – what about shopping for vegetables in the local market as opposed to the supermarket? Can you buy any of the basics for the baby second hand? This is especially useful for items that are only used for a short amount of time, such as the Moses basket, sling or sleep suits in the first three months. You need to take some control of the coming responsibility.

Many couples turn to the state for help in some areas. In addition to maternity benefit there is also child benefit and a range of options when it comes to childcare (see page 328, under parenthood support services, financial advice for parents). Some of these require complicated form filling, so it's best to work out what needs to be done in advance to avoid any last minute panics and the risk of losing out on something you may be entitled to claim.

your relationship

The arrival of a baby often prompts couples to look at their relationship. A much-wanted baby usually brings couples closer, but it can also highlight problem areas in a relationship. This is a good time to talk through any unresolved issues with your partner (and other children, if you have them). It is a good time to develop intimacy and forge closeness if you feel it is lacking.

I encourage couples to practise 'skin-to-skin' closeness (just as I encourage parents to do with infants), although I realize it's not for everyone. For those that prefer intimate talking, perhaps you can discuss how the baby will change the dynamic of your relationship (or relationships), the importance of fostering

family and friends game

Authors Judy Priest and Judith Schott[3] use buttons to demonstrate to parents-to-be the subtle but huge changes within relationships that the arrival of a baby can cause. You'll need a box of buttons or beads. Use one button to represent a friend, family member or a group of friends in your lives (for example, the gym friends). Choose a button to represent yourself, and a little button to represent the baby.

Place your buttons on a table around the button representing you in a pattern that you feel reflects your relationships with each person/group, placing those you spend most time with near the button representing you, and others further away. Think about the activities you do every week, and who is involved in them. Position your partner and his or her friends on the table, too.

Now place the baby in the middle of all this and think about how the dynamics will change. Who will you not be able to spend as much time with? Perhaps pub friends? Who will it be good to see more? Family and friends with children? This useful game can help you reassess relationships at any stage of life.

time together, and what this new addition will mean for the existing members. Perhaps plan a special weekend – or even a few weekends – for just the two of you before the baby comes (although make sure these weekends are before 37 weeks – you don't want to find yourself going into labour while on a crofting holiday in Scotland).

telling your other children about the baby

It can be difficult to hide an early pregnancy from a child, not least because they can be masters at picking up things that they are not supposed to hear. It may be difficult, but my advice is to try not to tell them until you are clear of the 12-week scan. There are two reasons for this: first, if you miscarry you will have to explain that to your child, which may be very upsetting for both of you; second, they may accidentally blurt it out.

Some women find it helpful to wait until their tummy starts to show a little bump – it makes it easier to explain the concept of 'Mummy has a baby in her tummy'. I think it's helpful to spend some time talking to them about it, even if they don't fully understand. Perhaps introduce the subject and, if they show no interest, gently come back to it another time.

If your children are a little older, you can involve them by discussing how they can help Mummy when the new baby arrives. Perhaps suggest they can do a feed, if you choose to do any bottle feeds, or fetch nappies and wipes. You can even ask if they can think of any names – this usually throws up some interesting suggestions! I've heard a range of interesting offers, from 'Jesus' to 'Steaker'. Closer to the birth, or immediately after the birth, you can buy a toddler their own Moses basket, crib or pushchair for their dolly so that they can mimic what Mummy does.

I encouraged my children to touch my tummy, to feel their siblings kicking and to listen to the heartbeat when the midwife was there. You can invite them to put the gel on your tummy, come to the scans or to look at the little print out from the scans.

The interaction between siblings is crucial to their childhoods and, in some cases, can have more of an impact than relationships with parents. Research done by Professor Robert Winston for a BBC documentary[4] showed that second and subsequent children have a heightened understanding of competition or 'sibling rivalry'.

coping with more than one child

It is often said that the biggest leap is from one child to two (or three if you are expecting twins), and certainly I would back that from my own experience. My first baby was a huge shock, even though he was planned. Perhaps I had more to deal with than most because my son had a heart problem and needed hospital treatment for the first six months of his life, but there were other factors, too, that made it so profoundly shocking.

I was always someone who had been out – whether busy at work, socializing with friends or just simply enjoying reading the papers in a cafe. Suddenly the front door was firmly closed. I couldn't go anywhere without him, even to nip to the corner shop to buy milk. I felt a total loss of freedom. My house was messy, I was messy, and the amount I needed to do to care for this tiny being was constant – relentlessly so.

Then, only 21 months later, we had a wonderful surprise – my daughter. But rather than being used to the chaos of children, I found this even more of a bombshell. Now I couldn't even leave a room alone if they were together. I had to keep an eye on them both all the time. Going to the shops was an ordeal because most of my time was spent trying to keep an eye on the older one to make sure he didn't disappear. When the second one started to walk, they would go in opposite directions – you may have two arms, but you only have one body. I used to struggle to get them in the car: one would be rigid, the other screaming. Almost every mother of two has clocked up parking tickets purely on the basis that, in the rush back to the car before the meter runs out, one child will invariably scream, 'I need to do a poo poo!'

Amazingly enough, child three and four made it much easier. I totally surrendered. Our family was child-friendly and the way we managed our lives was with the children firmly at the centre. I became much better able to cope with a hysterical child and we all got on with it. And the more children we had, the more we could train the older ones to help.

The point to remember, if you're expecting your second or a subsequent baby and are wondering how you will cope, is that each mother finds her own way. It will be difficult at first, but once you have got to know your baby and have the lay of the land, you will learn how to make the dynamic in your family work.

the start of a new life

The miracle of conception really is a miracle. That split-second moment in which the cells of a new life spring from old cells is still a mystery to medical science. How does this fundamental act of life occur? Over the course of the first trimester, your miracle baby will grow exponentially. That tiny first dividing cell will be transformed into the kicking, hiccupping acrobat that you see on the monitor at your 12-week scan. This scan, at the end of the first trimester, may be the first time your partner has the chance to connect with the little thing growing inside you and to acknowledge the feeling of becoming a parent.

Understanding how your baby is developing from early on in your pregnancy will allow you and your partner to feel more connected with your baby. Take the time to imagine what is going on inside your body at each stage of development. Research pictures that give you a glimpse into that inner world that is, at the moment, your baby's universe. Connecting with your unborn child in this way helps you develop the empathy that you need to be a responsive, caring parent, and is also fascinating to most mums- and dads-to-be.

WEEKS 0–6: THE WOMB BECOMES A HOME

The power of attraction between one man and one woman has led to the most intimate stage of a relationship – the act of sex – which entangles the souls and bodies of two people, leading to the release of sperm. These tireless voyagers make their difficult journey through the cervix (the neck of the womb) into the uterus and up into the Fallopian tubes. The distance they travel is short – only 15cm – but hazardous, taking 10 to 20 hours. One victorious sperm penetrates an egg and the fusion of genetic material from one man and one woman is successful, creating a new, unique human being. Every baby made was the first to win the race.

The fertilized egg travels along the Fallopian tube for two to three days. Within this time there is rapid cell division and the fertilized egg begins to look like a raspberry. There are two groups of cells – one that will become the baby and one that will become the placenta. By day five, the fertilized egg, now known as a blastocyst, arrives at the uterus.

For one tiny blastocyst, the uterus is a vast place. The tiny collection of cells must now connect with the womb lining for nourishment, in order to survive.

Its outer covering cracks and the blastocyst attaches itself to the mother, and will be dependent entirely on her body throughout its life within the womb. It nestles into the warm womb lining, enjoying the rich nourishment that allows for rapid growth. During the next few weeks, it develops from a tiny collection of cells into an embryo.

The baby at five weeks is only 4mm long and looks like a see-through worm. At one end is the brain and, running from top to bottom is a nerve tube. Alongside this nerve tube, 33 to 34 tiny back bones are beginning to develop and are loosely held in position by muscles and soft tissues. The baby's face takes a very basic shape – the holes of the nostrils, eyes and mouth are clearly seen but as yet not recognizable as a human being.

At around six weeks, your little baby's heart, which is by now the size of a poppy seed, begins to beat to speed and rhythm. (Once this happens, the chance of miscarriage reduces significantly.) The little arms and legs are still tiny buds, just beginning to sprout. By this time your little baby will be the size of a grain of rice or a sunflower seed and is shaped like a tiny 'S'.

The embryo is by now cushioned by amniotic fluid in the sac that will house him or her for the rest of the pregnancy. Outside the sac the tissue that will become the placenta is forming and, at this stage, is larger than the embryo. (By the end of this trimester, the placenta will take over the role of feeding the baby through the umbilical cord, which is already in place.) By the end

a world in your womb

It might be helpful to picture this world of wonder in your womb as:

- ⊙ a little sea (amniotic fluid) which will remain around your baby throughout the pregnancy, cushioning her from the outside world and holding her gently within her sanctuary
- ⊙ a peninsula (the placenta) connecting your baby to the greater land mass

(mother); the placenta embeds into the uterus and forms the link between your baby and your body, allowing oxygen and nutrients to flow easily between the two of you
- ⊙ the life line (the umbilical cord) which, like a rope, allows your baby to move freely through the womb whilst constantly linked to you and receiving nutrients from the placenta.

of the sixth week, eye lenses are beginning to form, as are the lungs, intestines and the urinary system.

WEEKS 6–8: RAPID CHANGE

This is an important time for the embryo: the major organs are developing, including the kidneys, gall bladder, lungs and pancreas. Intestines start to form within the umbilical cord that later become part of your baby's abdomen. The spine is also taking shape, as well as facial features: creases are forming where the eyelids will be as well as the tip of the nose, finger buds and the outline of toes. The hormone-producing glands, such as the pituitary, thyroid and adrenal glands, are beginning to take shape.

Your baby is taking on an increasingly human shape. By the seventh or eighth week the baby becomes a 'foetus' as opposed to an 'embryo'. By now, your baby is 5–10mm (measured from the top of the head to the bottom – the crown to rump length). Her fingers start to develop, as do little feet, which are webbed like duck feet. During this time, your baby will make the first jolts that, later on in pregnancy, you will feel as 'kicks' that make you realize you have an independent little person within your womb.

By week eight, your baby's head is huge in comparison to her body. She is swimming within her swimming pool and exercising her muscles and joints.

WEEKS 9–11: GOODBYE EMBRYO, HELLO BABY

Your chance of miscarriage is greatly reduced again once you pass eight weeks. The baby's heart is thumping at between 120 and 160 beats per minute.

During this time your baby's cartilage, bones, fingers and thumb are forming as well as the genitals, although you won't be able to tell the sex on an ultrasound scan. Further facial details are forming such as the upper lips, teeth and taste buds and a palate. The ear lobes are also beginning to take shape.

The major organs continue to develop at a pace and by the end of this time your baby has elbows and wrists, knees and ankles. By 10 weeks your baby is fully made and resembles a human being in tiny proportions. He is now 2–3cm long and weighs 10–15g (the weight of a small letter). He can skip, float and enjoy movement in his vast sea.

His brain is growing rapidly and has bones forming loosely over its surface so that it has the flexibility to expand freely. The umbilicus, the essential life line between mother and baby, has three vessels for blood flow – two arteries

ultrasound scan

In the UK, 10 to 12 weeks is the usual time for the first ultrasound scan (see page 56), allowing you to see and marvel at your amazing little baby on the screen, looking like a 'little kidney bean'. Within the womb you can see the heart beating rapidly, his little backbone, arms and legs, and his big head. You may even see your baby jumping on the screen.

(carrying deoxygenated blood away from the baby) and one vein (carrying oxygenated blood to the baby). The baby's toes are now looking more separate as webbing recedes. His hands are clearly seen with little fingers. His eyes are covered now by skin in the form of eyelids.

By the end of the trimester, your baby will be fully formed, with eyes and ears, nostrils, hands, feet, toes, the beginnings of fingernails and even hair. All of his major organs, including the brain, are in place and the vocal chords begin to form. He or she is about the size of your thumb.

By 12 weeks you can sometimes hear your baby's heartbeat with a hand-held Doppler when your midwife places it on your abdomen.

Your baby is very active now and, although you won't be able to feel anything, you may catch him somersaulting, hiccupping, boxing or 'dancing' when you have your ultrasound scan.

your antenatal care

To women pregnant for the first time, the system of antenatal care can seem a confusing mystery. Finding out what to expect and what kind of care you are entitled to will give you more confidence to get what you want from the health-care system during pregnancy and birth. I like to give the women I look after as much information as possible, to allow them to make the right personal choices for their intensely personal experience within the world of maternity care. This often makes women feel empowered and much more positive about the system they suddenly find themselves in. Thinking ahead to the birth, I advise you to read part two of this book at least once during each trimester. The information there will help you start planning and preparing for the kind of birth you want to have, explains how best to get your antenatal care providers to help you achieve that, and will also give you a good understanding of the childbirth process.

getting an early hospital referral

It's important to get an early hospital referral because the referral books you a bed. It is a good safety net, even if you think you may change your mind about where you want to give birth later (for choices of where to give birth, see pages 178–82). Even if you are booking a private obstetrician in a private hospital or private wing of an NHS hospital, you can't hang around. Private obstetricians usually also work in the NHS so only have a set number of places for private patients. They are predominantly based in London and they can book up as quickly, if not more quickly than NHS hospitals – especially if you are after an obstetrician who is well-known. (That said, an obstetrician with a particular specialization may take you on if, say, you discover something at your 12 or 20 to 22 week scan which makes your case unusual.) If you want to book a home birth, you still need to register with your local hospital to access the team of midwives who look after women having their babies at home.

In theory you have a choice when it comes to booking the hospital, but in reality that is not always the case. If you don't get a bed at the hospital of your choice, don't take it personally. Hospitals now work to a certain capacity per month to maintain safety standards. You will get into a hospital, it may not be

reasons for an early scan

You may be referred for an early scan if:

- ⊙ you have previously suffered a miscarriage
- ⊙ you have previously had a preterm baby
- ⊙ you have a baby with abnormalities
- ⊙ you experience heavy bleeding
- ⊙ you are a private patient
- ⊙ there is a chance you are having twins or more – doctors can tell this if your tummy is measuring higher than normal or if you have had fertility treatment or a family history of multiples.

the nearest. You can appeal, but there is no guarantee the decision will be overturned. (I should add here that if you are 'high risk' you may be referred to a hospital that specializes in your particular area.)

It's worth remembering that busy NHS hospitals, particularly those in cities, book up very quickly, so see your GP as soon as possible. Once booked, your NHS hospital will send you an appointment letter and a form to fill in. Your first appointment at the hospital will be when you are around 10 to 12 weeks pregnant. Here begins your 'episode of care'. (If you want to see someone before you are 12 weeks pregnant for any reason, other care providers are contactable through the Association of Early Pregnancy Units (see page 328 for contact details). An EPU can provide pregnancy testing, early ultrasound scans and access to doctors, nurses, midwives and support staff.)

For more information on where to give birth, private obstetricians and private midwives, see pages 178–82.

early scanning, pros and cons

Early scanning for non-urgent reasons is, like many areas in pregnancy, the subject of debate. Many private doctors recommend it, especially for women who are over 30. Other doctors argue that a misleading result can cause unnecessary upset and heartache. Many believe that unnecessary and frequent scanning is not a good trend. Everyone is encouraged to have a 12-week scan on the NHS as, by this time, the information is much easier to determine.

One of the obvious pros of an early scan is that you will find out if you are having more than one baby. It can also be reassuring – if after eight weeks there is a normal heartbeat, your chance of miscarriage is reduced to 3%.

However, unless there is good reason, you will usually have to have an early scan privately, which can cost up to £150. If you are unsure of your dates and you scan too early the results can also be misleading: the baby is tiny at this stage and it can be hard to get definite information.

If there is no foetal heartbeat visible you will usually be asked to return for a follow-up scan within two weeks. This can be a distressing wait. The follow-up scan, which you will also have to pay for, may show that you have had a 'missed miscarriage', or it may show the presence of a heartbeat and a normal foetus.

your first hospital appointment

Government recommendations are that your hospital appointment (the so-called 'booking' or 'booking in' appointment) takes place within 12 weeks of pregnancy – although obviously your GP needs to have referred you at least two weeks before, so make sure you see your GP in good time.

You need to be on time for your appointment, so leave with plenty of time in hand. In big, busy maternity units you may be at your appointment for as long as three hours. You will be checked in and then you will see a midwife. This may even be the first time you have met with a midwife. She will:

- ask you to provide a urine sample
- take your blood to test your:
  - blood group
  - RH factor (rhesus negative or positive, see page 66)
  - haemoglobin level
  - rubella (German measles) antibody level
  - exposure to venereal infection, such as syphilis, hepatitis B
  - exposure to HIV (you will be asked for your permission before your blood is tested for the HIV virus)
- weigh and measure you – from which she will calculate your BMI (see the information on pages 64–5)
- ask you for details of your medical history, your ongoing pregnancy, your partner's medical history and family history on both sides. This can take some time.

Your 'booking in' visit will determine what obstetric risks you may have – this could be to do with an existing medical condition or with something that comes up in this appointment.

At the end, you will be put into one of two categories:

⊙ low risk – if you are 'low risk', your pregnancy will be managed under normal midwife-led care or a combination of your GP and the hospital midwives
⊙ high risk – if you are 'high risk', you will be under the care of midwives, obstetricians and/or other specialists depending on your requirements. (For a list of what determines 'high risk, see page 62.)

For women who have complicated medical conditions, such as heart disease or diabetes, pregnancy can pose a number of complex concerns. You may be allocated a team of specialists who focus both on you (maternal medicine) and the baby (foetal medicine).

The majority of women will then have an ultrasound, which will be performed by a sonographer. Your sonographer may also be a qualified obstetrician or midwife.

the 12–week scan

This screening scan is done between 11 and 13 weeks and is only a guide – it cannot tell you for sure whether your baby has a chromosomal abnormality such as Down's syndrome (also known as trisomy 21; this condition causes delays in the way a baby grows and can affect the baby both mentally and physically). It is sometimes called the '12-week scan', 'the nuchal scan' or 'the combined test', depending on where you go. Different hospitals screen for different markers in this scan, usually done at around three months, but they are all, essentially, gauging the same thing – the probability of your baby having Down's syndrome.

The scan will usually be done in conjunction with a blood test that checks the level of Pregnancy Associated Placental Protein-A (PAPP-A) and Beta Human Chorionic Gonadotrophin (b-HCG). Low PAPP-A and high b-HCG can indicate Down's syndrome. The specialists then factor in your age as the risk of Down's syndrome increases with age. For example a woman of 25 has a 1:1000 chance, a woman of 35 has a 1:365 chance and a woman of 45 has a 1:32 chance.

Medical staff will determine your own personal ratio based on information from the scan, your blood test and your age. They will give you a result presented as a one in x number 'chance'.

Although the 12-week scans are now routine in this country, they are not compulsory. If you are going ahead with these tests you need to look at both sides of the outcome and ask yourself this – if there is a chance you may be carrying a baby with Down's syndrome, what will you do? Roughly 1 in 1,000 babies born in the UK have Down's syndrome. See page 327 for sources of information, advice and support.

Most hospitals will charge you a few pounds for a print out of your scan. All being well, you will probably leave your hospital appointment with a black and white picture of your baby in your hand and the first trimester behind you.

For some women their first hospital appointment is real confirmation that they are pregnant and this can give rise to many questions, hopes, plans and also fears.

further testing

If further tests are required, there are a number of tests available to check for abnormalities – screening tests and diagnostic tests. A screening test will tell you the chance of your baby having an abnormality, while a diagnostic test will tell you definitively whether your baby has one.

A screening test is safer and relies on the experience and expertise of the specialist who is examining. For example, in the case of the integrated test (see below) the examiner will look at the measurement of the nuchal fold (an area of skin on the back of your baby's neck) and then factor in your age and the results of a special blood test. Your result will appear as a probability, for example, 'Mrs Grey has a one in 500 chance of having a baby with Down's syndrome'. The only way Mrs Grey will know for certain that her baby actually has Down's syndrome in advance of the baby being born is to take a diagnostic test, such as CVS (see below) or an amniocentesis (see pages 121–2). These tests are both invasive, which means the doctor has to go in and extract tissues or fluid from around the baby that is then tested. These tests come with a risk of miscarriage.

NICE guidance

The National Institute of Clinical Excellence (NICE) is an independent body with the central aim of promoting good health and good health practice in the UK. NICE produces guidelines on public health, the use of medicine, treatment and procedure and on clinical practice. Hospital trusts refer to NICE when drawing up their own policies and guidelines.

All areas of pregnancy, birth and postnatal care are covered by NICE, including guidelines on induction, intrapartum care and Caesarean section. If you have any concerns about your condition or the care you are receiving you can check what guidelines NICE has set out for good practice. For sources of more information on NICE, see page 327.

FURTHER SCREENING TESTS IN THE FIRST TRIMESTER

The integrated test (see below) is embarked on during the first trimester. Depending on your hospital, the combined test (see pages 120–1) is carried out at 11 weeks plus five days or 13 weeks plus five days.

The integrated test is generally considered the best screening for Down's syndrome as it measures the nuchal fold and provides blood screening on four markers. The test is done in two parts. The first is the scan described above (between 11 and 13 weeks) to measure the nuchal fold at the back of your baby's neck. A blood sample is also taken to measure the concentration of pregnancy associated plasma protein.

The second part is done at 15 to 16 weeks (but not later than 22 weeks). There is also a further blood test, which looks at four markers (these are alpha-fetoprotien, free b-human chorionic gonadotrophin, unconjugated oestriol and inhibin-A. In pregnancies with Down's, PAPP-A and AFP tend to be low, and inhibin and freeb-HCG tend to be raised. The results then take into account all measurements, together with your age, to give you an estimation of your risk of having a baby with Down's syndrome. If you have a risk estimated at 1 in 150 you will be offered an amniocentesis (see pages 121–2).

CHORIONIC VILLUS SAMPLING (CVS)

This test, carried out between 10 and 13 weeks, is an alternative to amniocentesis and involves a small sample of tissue being taken from the edge of the placenta (chorion), using the ultrasound scan for guidance. From this sample, doctors can test for Down's syndrome and other chromosomal abnormalities, hereditary disorders, muscular dystrophy and haemophilia. The test takes around 20 minutes. The doctor will insert a needle through your abdomen to take the tissue sample.

I had this test myself in two pregnancies. I remember it as being quick but very intense. The advantage of CVS over amniocentesis is that if you decide to terminate the pregnancy, it can be done earlier. It is sensible to take someone with you if you are going to have this test.

twins and multiples

Perhaps you have twins in your family, perhaps you have a back-of-the-mind inkling that there may be more than one in there, perhaps you have had fertility treatment and are aware that there may be more than one. As you get older, your body can release more than one egg when you ovulate, which means you have an increased chance of conceiving twins. Statistics show that you have a 3% chance if you are aged between 25 and 29, 4% between the ages of 30 and 34 and almost 5% if you are aged between 35 and 39.

Whatever your reasons, yours may be one of the many multiples in the UK. Regardless of your chances, for most women it still feels like a totally unexpected shock. It will take some time to absorb the news and many women go through a lot of emotions when they discover they are carrying twins. You may be thinking, 'Oh my goodness: the money, the tiredness, the double-sized bump – how will I cope?' You may also be thinking, 'Hey, how fantastic: one pregnancy, two babies! They will entertain themselves, they will have a wonderful bond.'

Certainly there is double the fabulousness when you are expecting two. There are so many positives. Knowing you are carrying two babies means that, right from the start, you know your path will be different from your friends with only one baby. Automatically you will be labelled as a 'high-risk' case and you will probably be facing a birth with more medicalization than if you were only carrying one.

identical and non-identical twins

Non-identical (dichorionic) twins are conceived from two separate eggs fertilized by two separate sperm. They develop in their own amniotic sacs with their own placentas. They can be the same sex or a boy and a girl.

Identical twins (monochorionic) are conceived from one egg and one sperm. Because their genetic material is identical they are, obviously, always the same sex and occur in one in three twin births. Monochorionic and dichorionic can be diagnosed as early as eight weeks, but it's not always possible to diagnose identical twins on a 20-week ultrasound scan, and there are a number of complex reasons for this:

⊙ you may not be able to see the sex of both babies
⊙ sometimes in an identical twin conception the egg splits early in the pregnancy – between day 7 and day 14. This results in separate sacs and separate placentas
⊙ in some cases the placentas of non-identical twins fuse into one causing a misdiagnosis between monochorionic and dichorionic.

Because twins are never straightforward, it is also possible to have identical twins who do not look alike. This happens when the two babies don't have equal access to the same amount of nutrients from their shared placenta, perhaps because of how they are lying in the womb. In this situation one baby grows faster and bigger than the other. Their weight at birth may be dramatically different and, although weight will usually equalize later, the difference in the way the babies look in the face or body may remain for life.

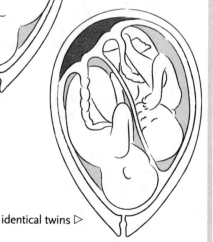

◁ non-identical twins

identical twins ▷

In other respects, too, you will need to be more aware. You will need to take even more care of yourself than a mother with one baby and you will probably find that you show earlier. You will have an extenuation of the 'minor disorders' such as back pain, indigestion, swelling in the legs, heartburn and breathlessness, and you may also be more prone to iron deficiency.

One thing is certain, twins is double the work at the beginning and you can't be shy on recruiting everyone you can possibly think of for help. You will also need to think seriously about giving up work earlier as today, doctors like to deliver twins at around 37 weeks. The Caesarean section rate is much higher with twins – usually around 50% compared with 23% for normal pregnancies, because of the risk to the second twin.

At Queen Charlotte's hospital, all monochorionic twins (identical twins, see opposite) are delivered by Caesarean section. In addition, a Caesarean will be recommended for any pregnancy where the first twin is not 'head down', and in the case of any twin pregnancies where the mother goes into premature labour.

Having said all that, I do have experience with mothers who have had 'natural' deliveries with twins. I helped look after one mother who was pregnant with twins. Both babies were 'head down' almost side by side. She went into spontaneous (not induced) labour at 40 weeks. When she arrived at the hospital she was 4cm dilated and we used intermittent monitoring with hand-held Dopplers as opposed to constant CTG monitoring with a machine. Because the babies' backs were on opposite sides, the separate heartbeats were distinctive – and both thumping along at different rates.

She decided to stand to deliver the first baby, and was carrying this baby and kneeling down to deliver the second. She delivered both placentas naturally and, although the babies weighed over 3kg (6.5lb) each, she needed no stitches. So it can be done. See page 327 for sources of information and support organizations for families with twins.

early pregnancy complications

Most women have straightforward pregnancies, but in some cases, things become complicated. In such cases, the more information a woman has, the better able she is to take care of herself and her baby, deal with difficult situations, and make the right choices for herself for a healthy outcome.

HIGH-RISK PREGNANCY

You are considered high risk and will be monitored more closely during your pregnancy, if you:

- are over 40 years old and having your first baby
- are having a multiple pregnancy (i.e. twins, triplets etc)
- suffer from high blood pressure
- are obese (if you have a BMI above 35 you will be assigned an obstetrician)
- are addicted to drugs or alcohol
- previously had a preterm baby (a baby born before 37 weeks)
- previously had a baby with an abnormality
- have had a previous Caesarean – there is a 0.5% risk of a rupture of the muscle in the lower uterus
- suffer from a serious illness or a condition such as diabetes, epilepsy, a heart condition, thyroid or kidney problems, or have cancer or HIV
- take heavy medication, such as anti-psychotic drugs
- have any mental health problems
- are in your teens
- are socially deprived.

When you see your GP in the very early weeks, make sure you give them a full and complete medical history. You will also be asked about your medical history at your booking appointment at the hospital.

MISCARRIAGE

Doctors today believe that 15% of known pregnancies result in miscarriage. The rate for women over 40 rises to 25%. The vast majority of these are in the very early weeks.

If you do experience a miscarriage, don't blame yourself or think 'what did I do wrong?' Anywhere between 40% and 75% of early miscarriages are thought to be as a result of a chance chromosomal abnormality in the embryo or foetus that is unlikely to re-occur. The chances of miscarriage as a result of a chromosomal abnormality do, however, increase with maternal age.

Some women feel comforted by the idea that this is 'nature taking its course', in the knowledge that the baby would not have been able to survive pregnancy or birth. Others want to know exactly what caused the miscarriage to ensure it will not be a recurrent problem. If you have two miscarriages you are at higher risk of having a third. If you have three, you will be referred to a specialist. If you have already had two miscarriages and then fall pregnant, you may be told to take certain precautions, such as avoiding sex, especially around the time you would have had your period. You may also be advised to avoid flying.

If you experience any 'spotting' (spots of brownish blood in your knickers), bleeding, or a complete loss of pregnancy symptoms, let your doctor know. However, don't forget that many women do have spotting as part of a normal pregnancy. Heavy bleeding, especially with blood clots, is obviously a concern, and you should alert your doctor immediately. Not all women miscarry in this way and some only discover they have miscarried when they are scanned and there is no foetal heartbeat. This is called a 'missed miscarriage'. The doctor may offer you what used to be called a D&C (dilation and curettage), but is now often referred to as an ERPC (evacuation of retained products of conception), an operation to remove the failed pregnancy. Some women, however, prefer to wait and to let 'nature take its course'. This can take a few weeks.

At 10 weeks the chance of miscarriage drops to 15% and, by 12 weeks, the chances of miscarrying are no more than 1% (although this does not guarantee everything is perfect).

If you have opted for the private route and have an early scan at six or eight weeks, the consultant carrying out the scan may see a foetal heartbeat. Statistics

the risk of miscarriage

According to research by the children's charity Tommy's, the relative risk of miscarriage is as follows:

⊙ first pregnancy 5%
⊙ last pregnancy a live birth 5%
⊙ two or more previous pregnancies resulted in live birth 4%
⊙ one previous miscarriage 20%
⊙ two previous miscarriages 28%
⊙ three previous miscarriages 43%.

show that an eight-week-old foetus with a heartbeat has a 97% chance of going full-term as a healthy pregnancy.

It can be an immensely stressful experience, particularly with a much wanted, much tried for baby. For support, advice and help after a miscarriage, contact the Miscarriage Association (for contact details, see page 328).

ECTOPIC PREGNANCY

An ectopic pregnancy occurs when the egg is fertilized and implants somewhere other than the uterus, for example the Fallopian tube, the ovary, the abdomen or the scar of a previous Caesarean section.

You may still have a positive pregnancy test result, even though in most cases it is not a viable pregnancy. Most ectopic pregnancies are diagnosed between the sixth and seventh week of pregnancy and the symptoms can include serious abdominal pain, shoulder tip pain and abdominal bleeding. Report any such symptoms to your doctor immediately.

Approximately 1% of women experience an ectopic pregnancy. Although all sexually active women of childbearing age are at risk of an ectopic pregnancy, those who have fertility treatment are believed to be at slightly higher risk.

Research shows that you may also be at more risk if you have had pelvic inflammatory disease, endometriosis, any abdominal surgery (including a Caesarean section), or if you have had a coil fitted or were on the progesterone-only contraceptive pill (mini pill). Surgery is usually required to end the pregnancy and prevent any further complications.

See page 328 for sources of further information on ectopic pregnancy.

OBESE AND UNDERWEIGHT MOTHERS

Your BMI is a calculation made by dividing your weight with the square of your height. The result is then charted in a range of underweight, normal, overweight or obese. The method of calculating a person's health based on their BMI is now routine in the NHS, particularly in the wake of health fears linked to the rise of obesity. It also has a place in pregnancy. Most women are weighed between 10 and 12 weeks at their hospital booking appointment, but if you have any concerns about your weight, make sure you see your GP as soon as possible. While BMI it is a useful tool for women who start pregnancy either very underweight or obese (see below), I will say here that I believe it can also be misleading for those with normal weight. In general, if you have a BMI between

20 and 25, and you are eating normally, you should not need to be weighed throughout pregnancy.

MOTHERS WHO ARE OVERWEIGHT It's more difficult to gauge the position, size and lie of the baby when the mother is carrying excess weight on her stomach. It is also more difficult to determine accurate measurements on the ultrasound. Women with a BMI of above 25 are more likely to have heavier babies and around half give birth by Caesarean section. They often need to wear larger blood pressure cuffs and some hospitals have introduced special beds and surgery tables for women who weigh up to and over 30 stones (190kg).

If you are overweight or obese at the start of your pregnancy, you are at a much greater risk of miscarriage, having dangerously high blood pressure, clots, diabetes and heart disease, and you are more prone to bleeding. As a result, women who are overweight or obese also have a greater risk of maternal death[5] and may also have an increased risk of babies with birth defects[6] and stillbirth.[7]

It is very important to get help as early as possible. Make sure you are referred to a nutritionist and that your weight is closely monitored.

MOTHERS WHO ARE UNDERWEIGHT Equally problematic for pregnancy is a BMI measurement of less than 18.5. In addition to feeling the minor disorders more acutely, mothers who are underweight are more likely to find it harder to cope with pregnancy. Pregnancy itself can also exacerbate the underlying condition that causes low weight in the first place – such as an eating disorder or drug problem.

The implications are perhaps most worrying for the baby. A mother-to-be with a very low BMI usually delivers a low-birth-weight baby and this can affect the baby's ability to feed and grow for up to six months after birth. The baby is also at increased risk of complications such as hypothermia, low blood sugar and viral infections.

Women with eating disorders such as anorexia nervosa or bulimia need to be treated by a psychiatrist, in addition to the care they receive from their doctor and obstetrician.

However, as 2% of women are now thought to develop eating disorders during pregnancy,[8] it is also essential that you speak up if you are concerned about your weight or about putting on weight during the pregnancy.

See page 327 for sources of support for people with eating disorders.

RHESUS NEGATIVE MOTHERS

If you are rhesus negative (RhD neg) and your baby is rhesus positive (RhD pos), your doctor will want to ensure that none of the baby's blood will mix with yours. If that happens, your body will produce antibodies to fight what it assumes to be a foreign invader.

There are a number of situations that may put your baby's blood in contact with yours in the early weeks, including ectopic pregnancy, vaginal bleeding or diagnostic tests such as CVS or amniocentesis. During birth, there is a very high risk your baby's blood will come into contact with yours.

To prevent your body producing antibodies, you will be given an ante d prophylaxis by injection in the thigh if you are at risk in the early weeks or routinely between 28 and 34 weeks, unless there is a specific reason why you don't want or need it. If you know your partner is definitely RhD negative, you do not require ante d prophylaxis. If you have any concerns, speak to your doctor or midwife.

RUBELLA

Rubella is caused by the rubella virus, which is extremely contagious and can be caught from coughs and sneezes. All women are checked for their rubella immunity at their booking appointment at the hospital. If you are not immune your baby is at risk so it is very important that you stay away from anyone who has the virus, because if you get rubella in the first trimester before 10 weeks there is a 90% chance that your baby will be affected with congenital brain damage, deafness, heart defects or cataracts. If you get rubella during the second trimester, the baby may develop sight and hearing problems and, during the third trimester, the risk is low.

If you do come into contact with someone who has rubella, you must contact your GP or obstetrician immediately. You will be strongly advised to have the MMR vaccine following the birth of your baby.

PRENATAL DEPRESSION

Prenatal depression is an under-researched area that is gaining recognition. It is now thought that as many as 70% of women have periods of feeling 'blue' in their pregnancies, and 10–15% suffer severely, feeling 'very black'. In part, depression may be caused by the enormous surge in hormones that can make you feel 'not yourself'. It may also be caused by outside factors such as a complicated domestic or work situation, or stress.

A common symptom in the first trimester is 'feeling very alone' and this may be partly because many women don't tell friends and colleagues that they are pregnant until the beginning of the second trimester. If that feeling of loneliness begins to be overwhelming, it is important to speak up. Share the feelings with your partner, a friend or a medical professional.

I believe another reason why women can sink into a terrible low is if they are not getting any rest and cannot cope with the immense tiredness. The two can compound – a woman who is feeling depressed may be less good at looking after herself. The potent combination of hunger, nausea and exhaustion can also push some women further into a slump. They may start to alienate themselves. Some women describe their depression as 'like disappearing into a black hole' and 'waking up and just feeling terrible that I had to face another day'. Others talk of 'cycles' of depression and 'crying all the time'.

Women who smoke and are using alcohol or drugs are at higher risk of prenatal depression and need to get help. If you have a previous history with depression or any associated disorder, it's vital that you mention this as soon as possible to your GP, as well as at your hospital booking appointment. Don't wait for your hospital booking appointment if you're feeling overwhelmed. See your GP and get referred to someone who can help. This is hugely important as prenatal depression often strikes long before your first hospital appointment.

For some women the depression can be comparatively mild and be greatly eased by a combination of tailored care and counselling. For others, the depression is severe and medical treatment is recommended. If you have thoughts of suicide you need to get help urgently – if you can't get hold of your midwife or doctor, call Samaritans (see page 327 for contact details). Most cases of pregnancy-related depression lift after the first trimester, but in some cases they can continue throughout and may need ongoing treatment.

mental health problems and pregnancy

If you are taking medication to treat an existing mental health problem, continue with your prescription but see your doctor and psychiatrist as soon as you discover you are pregnant.

preparing your mind for birth

The mind can be a powerful tool. People who face and overcome extraordinary challenges against the odds (such as mountaineers and survivors of disasters) often claim that their minds worked just as hard as their bodies to help them achieve success.

For most women, childbirth is considered one of the most challenging experiences of a woman's life, and in my experience, women who have undertaken appropriate mental preparation in advance of their births have a far more enjoyable birth outcome. However, to prepare your mind for birth, you do have to put some work in beforehand.

First, you must challenge and dispel any fears you have about childbirth that

the fear-tension-pain cycle

Dr Grantly Dick-Read (1890–1959) was a British consultant obstetrician, who completely changed his thinking on childbirth after witnessing a young woman giving birth naturally with an old woman by her side. The woman's words to him afterwards were, 'It didn't hurt. It wasn't meant to was it Doctor?'

From here Dick-Read developed the idea of the relationship between fear, tension and pain in childbirth as a downward spiral. In addition to noting the obvious (that women who were terrified of birth had thoroughly unpleasant experiences) he also noticed the counter argument – that those who were calm and accepting seemed to feel less pain. They let their natural endorphins wash over them and seemed

at peace, even when the contractions were quite intense.

Grantly Dick-Read published his findings in *Childbirth Without Fear* in 1944.[9] This book was met with international acclaim and is still in print today. He makes it clear, however, that pain relief may be required for women undergoing abnormal labour – it was not his intention that the pain of labour should be unbearable. His philosophy was that women and society as a whole should approach natural birth positively, and without unnecessary medical intervention from obstetricians. He was the first president of the Natural Childbirth Trust, which went on to become the National Childbirth Trust (NCT).

are based on the negative popular myths about birth that abound in our society, despite the fact that women have been giving birth for millennia. Excessive (and unnecessary) fears about birth can have a negative impact themselves on your birth experience (see Fear–tension–pain cycle, opposite). Then you need to develop an armoury of mental tools that can help you through your birth experience and, by starting this task now, in your first trimester, you will give yourself ample time to do so.

negative myths about childbirth

Sadly, the common portrayal of birth in films and on television soap operas, is of a woman lying flat on her back, her privacy exposed to the world, screaming her head off with a chorus of relatives cheerleading her to 'push'. It's a ridiculous image and one, thank goodness, that is very rarely seen in real life. Only in huge emergencies, when the baby has to come out at great speed, is birth anything like this. Even then, it's only for a matter of minutes.

Dramas, in order to be just that, need to reinforce this skewed perception of birth as a terrifying and excruciating experience. However, it only really serves to scare women about birth and make most think that they need to reach for the epidural needle even before labour has started.

In order to get over the hump that is a stereotyped view of birth, women need to start thinking about their ideal birth. I always suggest reading some positive birth stories and talking to friends or colleagues who have enjoyed the experience. It may also help to ask those who have negative stories to tell what they would do differently a second time around. Finally you can ask your midwife about the births she has been present at – are there any memorable ones she can share with you? Why were they so amazing? How had that mother prepared for her birth? Inform yourself as much as possible about what really happens during labour and birth to get a realistic perspective.

'I had my second and third babies with Jenny and they were amazing in different ways. For my first birth I had an epidural, so second time around I wanted to try for natural. Some people would say that I was just lucky to have three easy labours and, yes, I am. But I did a lot of preparation. I went swimming every day. I read A LOT – Michel Odent, Gowri Motha, Ina May Gaskin – and took the information on board and really tried to connect with what was happening. I also used the Maggie Howell's natal hypnotherapy CD that I now recommend to everyone. I listened to the CD religiously. I really paid attention to Michel Odent's stuff about being in the dark and in a safe place and found that really powerful.

And of course, Ina May Gaskin's Spiritual Midwifery was an amazing inspiration. She makes you realize you are in control of your body and that you can visualise yourself opening like a flower and imagine and help your baby along if you have the self belief.

Whenever I thought I might hit an issue, I put the work in. Joseph was breech until 36 weeks. I got on all fours and cleaned the floors, I went swimming, I looked at tons of websites about how to get your baby into the best position and did a lot of talking to him, and he turned.

Louisa was a home birth so I wanted to make sure I didn't have one of those 24-hour labours. I was obsessive about getting the baby into a good position – every time I watched TV I was bouncing on the birth ball. During one of the checks Jenny noticed that the baby had her little hand on her head so I talked to the baby and asked her to move her hand down and she moved into the right position.

I had great labours, yes, but I did the mental preparation for them – I really believe it was worth it.' **GEORGIA, 35**

(For information on the books Georgia mentions, see suggested further reading, page 329. For sources of information on Maggie Howell's natal hypnotherapy, see page 329.)

visualisation as a mental tool

I am a firm believer (and I should be, having seen the results) in using 'visualisation' to help women get through labour and birth. A visualisation can be described as something like a day dream, a mental short film that you play in your head that allows you to imagine a desired outcome or side-step the negative sensations of the immediate situation you are in by mentally transporting yourself to a situation that nourishes your energy rather than depletes it.

Most famously, athletes (but also, many people from all walks of life) use visualisation to boost mental strength in challenging situations. Psychologists explain that the nature of your thoughts, be they positive or negative, has an impact on your state of mind and, consequently, your body. Positive thoughts, leading to a positive mental state, can produce powerful results.

For example, repeatedly imagining a wished-for outcome (scoring that tricky goal, reaching the peak of that impossible mountain) trains the brain to believe that it can be done – in a sense by 'tricking' the brain into believing that it has been done through the repeated conjuring of a mental picture. The brain 'tells' the body it can be achieved and 'allows' the body to achieve the desired result. Developing a detailed visualisation of a 'safe zone' to escape into can allow people to cope with physically and mentally challenging situations much more effectively, by allowing them some respite from the difficulties they face and nourishing their mind, body and soul during the difficulties when, without them, they might simply be more depleted by them.

I strongly advise that you develop your own personal visualisation over the coming months to help you through your experience of labour and birth.

> ## mantras for pregnancy
>
> It may help you to post the following positive thoughts on your computer, bathroom mirror, fridge or wherever you will see them regularly:
>
> 'Be positive'
> 'Everything will be fine'
> 'Patience, patience'
> 'Stay calm'
> 'Stay on top of things'.

MAKING THE HEAD STRONGER THAN THE UTERUS
By this, I mean making the power of your mind stronger than the power of a

contraction. If you can do this, you may well be able to enjoy your childbirth experience. This is where visualisation comes in.

The visualisation can be connected to the situation you are experiencing – perhaps even symbolic of it. For example, one of the most common visualisations during labour is to picture the contraction as a wave crashing against a shore and then retreating, taking with it shingle and sand. You may prefer complete detachment, for example an escape to the memory of a favourite beach holiday or spring walk in the countryside, taking in all the details of the birds, flowers, grass and trees, to make you feel calm and serene. Many people find the repetition of their visualisations work well in combating the repetition of the contractions.

I suggest that you start practising visualisation techniques now, even this far ahead of the big event, so that they are almost automatic when the time comes. There is no reason why your visualisations shouldn't help you in these early weeks of pregnancy, especially if you are struggling with the trials of such hormonal turmoil at a time when you are not supposed to tell anyone.

establishing your own visualisation

During the first trimester, start to develop a visualisation that you can expand on during your pregnancy. First, think of where you would most like to be in the world, a place you think is beautiful, where you feel nurtured by the environment. It could be a place where you holidayed as a child, your favourite park, your bed, a beach, a boat, or an imagined place. Once you know where you want your visualisation to be set, start to draw the scene in detail. Where are you sitting/lying? What can you see? Are there mountains in the distance, trees, a lake? Can you see the sky or sea?

Can you see the sun, moon or stars? A sunrise or a sunset? Draw the distance clearly in your mind. Now move closer to yourself. What is in your immediate surroundings? Grass, pebbles, a house, a tent, a little home-made fire, a winding path, a picnic, a tree, a pond? The idea is to make the scene as detailed as you can. Once you have a detailed 'view', return to it every day for 10 minutes. While you are sitting with your eyes closed, picturing your scene in detail, breathe deep out-breaths that reach your lower tummy. The deeper the out-breath, the deeper the relaxation.

MAKING A START Perhaps you could start by taking five minutes of each day to sit quietly and focus on building up a visualisation. Start by thinking about your growing baby, your changing body and this huge next step in your life. Embrace the physical changes, your growing tummy and breasts, and marvel at the incredible abilities of the human body. Then think about finding a visualisation that works for you (see the box opposite, to give you some ideas for how to get started).

learning patience

Time in the first trimester sometimes seems to stand still. Don't panic about how long it's taking – this is all good time for preparation. Start with the simple exercise of developing your patience in preparation for the birth. Everyone is always in a hurry – it's a modern-day malaise. There's no need to rush. When someone annoys you – a put-down at work, a queue barge at the post office, jumping lanes in the traffic – take a deep breath and, as you breathe out, breathe away the problem.

Patience is an essential tool of parenting. Everything that you learn now is an investment for the future. It's worth mentioning here that in some respects the trials of the first trimester mirror the first 12 weeks after birth: chronic tiredness, hormonal surges, a feeling of being vulnerable, super-sensitive and scatty. In some respects you have to surrender to these natural processes, in others, knowledge of what is happening to you will help you maintain control of your feelings and your life.

relaxation techniques

Teaching yourself to relax – and release – is an essential part of a happy, healthy pregnancy, of labour and for coping after the baby is born. You can use a variety of different techniques to aid relaxation.

TOUCH Ask your partner to place their hands firmly over the area that is holding tension, such as the back of your neck, shoulders, or the base of your spine. Light pressure in itself may be very soothing and you may appreciate pressure on your temples or forehead too. Perhaps close your eyes and take deep breaths as you relax into your partner's hands.

MASSAGE Massage is a step up from touch and should only be used very lightly by a non-professional to avoid causing any injury. As I said before, the ligaments soften and loosen during pregnancy and so you need to be especially careful that you don't attempt anything too hard.

Ask your partner to apply a light massage to the areas mentioned above – temples, neck, shoulders – as well as the upper arms, lower back, thighs and even the calves (but not the ankles), and gently on the feet.

WARM WATER During all my labours I insisted on a warm flannel over my face. It provided both a physical and symbolic barrier between my mind and the world and the weight and warmth of the flannel was also very relaxing on my face. It's a good one to try in the bath during pregnancy when you are very tired or want to relax.

A warm compress or hot water bottle wrapped in towels is also good for lower back pain, and a warm bath or shower trained on painful areas can greatly relieve tension in the shoulders, upper back, lower back and sacrum.

BREATH In addition to your mind, your breath is one of the most powerful weapons for combating tension, anxiety and the intensity of labour contractions. Slowing your breathing automatically makes you feel more relaxed and there are many other exercises that can help you reach a truly relaxed state.

Ask your partner to time how many breaths you take in 60 seconds when breathing normally. Then ask him to time you while you concentrate on breathing slowly – ideally you want to cut the number of breaths per minute in half. Try to count to five on the in-breath and seven or eight on the out-breath. Imagine breathing out all your anxieties and tension. This will be very useful for early labour. Another great technique that's worth practising for labour is a deep long breath in and then breathing out through your lips, as if you were blowing through a musical instrument.

THINGS TO THINK ABOUT

⊙ Look after yourself in pregnancy – even when you feel overwhelmed by hormones, you can still take charge and make a difference. I have given you advice from other mothers on how to cope – don't be afraid to try them out.

⊙ Build your mental strength – this is invaluable not just for pregnancy, but for life with small children.

⊙ It's never too early to think about the birth, where you want to give birth and with whom. Take some time to read the chapter Preparing your Birth Plan in part two (see pages 174–220) to find out what choices you have about where to give birth, and what kind of birth experience you would like. This will help you make a start on writing your birth plan. I recommend you read part two of this book at least once a trimester, and again just prior to birth, to help you prepare for your labour and birth. Don't forget to expect the unexpected. Start to build an idea of what you want in an ideal world, but also build an idea of your choices when things stray from the main plan.

⊙ Put some effort into researching your choices locally. Is the main hospital your only option for birth? Are there pregnancy yoga classes available near you? What else is on offer?

second trimester
13–26 weeks

The second trimester is generally considered to be the best in terms of the way you feel. Most women report a marked increase in energy, a calmer mood and, generally, a more positive outlook. The raging hormones of the first trimester are subsiding and it is easier to sleep, eat and get on with the day. Take advantage of this wonderful time. You can tell those around you that you are pregnant and they will probably comment on how fabulous you look. The most exciting part, perhaps, is that you will start to feel the baby moving.

coping with physical changes

The sickness and tiredness are abating and, although some women experience these symptoms until 16 weeks (or even longer), the majority of women will be putting the dark days of the first trimester behind them. Perhaps you will now be showing enough to be offered a seat on the train or bus. Maybe you are still in your old jeans and wondering when your bump is going to pop out. Everyone is different.

In addition to the feelings of wellbeing, there are a host of new possible pregnancy symptoms, some of which are welcome, such as that general 'pregnancy glow', thicker hair and a buoyant upbeat mood. Others, such as varicose veins, are less pleasant. It may be that you only experience very few, if any, of these signs. Again, everyone is different.

GLOWING COMPLEXION

What a relief to finally have a pregnancy symptom you can show off about! Your circulation increases by as much as 50% when you are pregnant, leaving you with a rosy complexion that's often referred to as the 'pregnancy glow'. In addition to the bloom caused by vasodilation (the dilation of blood vessels, caused by increased blood flow combined with the relaxing effect of progesterone), you may notice a slight sheen to your skin caused by an increase in oil secretions.

Of course oily secretions can also cause spots and rosy complexions can also be far more sensitive. You may find your skin reacting to harsher beauty products, particularly facial scrubs, and I recommend you go for the most simple, natural products available.

THREAD VEINS OR 'SPIDER VEINS'

Your increased circulation can also lead to thread veins, particularly on the legs. These appear as tiny red lines and may appear to spread as the pregnancy progresses. Most women find that they miraculously disappear very shortly after childbirth, although they can return with subsequent pregnancies. If they don't disappear after pregnancy and you are very conscious of them, they can be removed with a laser.

'PREGNANCY MASK'

Pregnancy hormones cause your body to produce more melanin (pigment), which is the substance that darkens your skin in the sun – and it shows in a number of ways. One is the 'pregnancy mask' (chloasma), a patchy darkening of the complexion, most noticeable on the forehead, nose, cheeks and around the lips, almost like lip-liner.

This is not a universal symptom and mostly affects women with darker complexions, but if you spend a lot of time in the sun, it may become more pronounced, as will freckles, some moles and birthmarks. Most pregnant women find they get a 'blotchy' tan because of the over-production of melanin.

DARKENING OF THE AREOLA

Melanin is also responsible for the darkening of the area around your nipples, or the areola. Birthmarks, too, can become deeper in colour and more pronounced. Some women, again, those with darker colouring, also notice dark circles around their eyes. Although in general your skin tone will return to normal after the birth, your areola may remain a shade darker than before.

LINEA NIGRA

This is another side effect of melanin. All women have a very fine, almost invisible white line (linea alba) that runs from their tummy button to their pelvic bone. In some women this line darkens during pregnancy and can even extend beyond the abdominal wall to the top of the bump. It will fade and disappear a few months after delivery and is nothing to be concerned about. Interestingly, doctors often use the presence of linea nigra to distinguish between a woman who is pregnant and a woman who has an ovarian cyst, although not every pregnant woman develops it.

NOTICEABLE CHANGES TO YOUR HAIR

Your hair may feel thicker as the pregnancy goes along, a symptom that delights those with fine hair and infuriates those with heavy locks. The reason for this is that the natural hair loss of everyday life slows during pregnancy, making your hair feel fuller and thicker. About three to five months after birth, some women experience what they often think is hair loss – they may even feel it is falling out in clumps. In the vast majority of cases, this is just the old hair falling out and new hair is growing in its place. If you feel it is more extreme than this, consult your doctor.

Your hair may also be drier or more greasy than normal, and some fairer women say their hair darkens during pregnancy. You may find that your hair reacts very differently to being coloured and turns a completely unexpected shade.

As I've said before, try to stick to products containing the least amount of chemicals that you can find for your skin and hair. Although my advice is to 'stay pure' (see pages 34–5), I realize that if you have been highlighting your hair for many years, the idea of leaving it to grow out, just at the point that your whole body is changing so dramatically, might be one 'natural' step too far. Do make sure, however, that your hairdresser knows that you are pregnant and avoids the scalp when applying any hair dye. Chemicals can enter the blood supply through your skin, which is why it is also best to avoid all beauty treatments, including fake tans.

'SKIN TAGS' AND RED DOTS

A skin change you may notice are little 'skin tags', often in the folds of your skin or in places where your clothes have rubbed. These are harmless and should disappear after the birth. If not, they can easily be removed. Some women also notice the random appearance of small red dots on the surface of the skin, like prickly heat (these are not similar to chicken pox or measles, which need to be reported to your GP). These are harmless and usually subside after pregnancy.

CONSTIPATION AND HAEMORRHOIDS

I discuss constipation, and tips for avoiding and relieving it on page 21. I mention constipation again here because straining when you are on the loo can increase your risk of haemorrhoids (piles). To reiterate, the bowel absorbs more fluid when you are pregnant, so you need to keep hydrated and include fibre and oils in your diet to help move food down the intestines more efficiently.

Half of all pregnant women experience haemorrhoids. Symptoms include rectal bleeding, itching and pain. If there is a family history of piles you may be more likely to get them. Equally, if you are already prone to constipation or irritable bowel syndrome, you may be more at risk. In the vast majority of cases, however, they clear up after pregnancy.

You can relieve the pain of haemorrhoids with cold gel pads, witch hazel or by using a sitz bath (otherwise known as a hip bath, in which only the hips and

haemorrhoids

Use the following tips to help you avoid haemorrhoids:

- ⊙ drink fluids – the bowel absorbs more fluid during pregnancy (drinking plenty of water will also make piles easier to manage)
- ⊙ include plenty of fibre and oil in your diet, such as dried apricots, figs and linseed pulp
- ⊙ avoid the temptation to strain when you go to the loo
- ⊙ avoid putting on too much weight
- ⊙ exercise – a brisk walk or swim is recommended
- ⊙ don't stand or sit in one position for too long
- ⊙ avoid 'bucket' seats and crossing your legs too much – where possible sit with your legs up on a stool or cushion
- ⊙ try to sleep on your side (left is best) – it takes the pressure off the affected veins
- ⊙ keep up with your pelvic floor exercises (see pages 37–8)
- ⊙ avoid heavy lifting
- ⊙ steer clear of knee-high tights
- ⊙ try to walk upright as much as you can rather than leaning either slightly forward or backward.

buttocks are soaked) filled with warm salted water. Acupuncture is effective as a preventative measure and Vitamin C is often recommended because it helps keep your veins 'elastic'. Topical ointments, such as Anusol, are also available, but check with your doctor or midwife before using any creams or laxatives.

VARICOSE VEINS

You may have noticed that all your veins are more prominent, including those on your chest, which may now resemble a road map. You may also have 'spider veins' appearing on your legs (see page 77). Veins have valves that allow the blood to keep pumping in one direction towards the heart. The pregnancy hormone progesterone causes the blood vessel walls to relax and the valves can fail or become incompetent. This causes blood to pool in places where gravity causes pressure – such as the legs – and can lead to varicose veins.

You may first notice varicose veins as swollen areas on your legs that start to itch. Your legs may also feel heavy and ache. The veins then darken and become more prominent, sometimes appearing like bulging knots. They can sting, ache, burn and itch furiously. They can even bleed and your ankles may also swell.

A popular treatment is support tights, which prop up the veins from the outside, stopping the blood from pooling. It also helps to make sure you are not standing or sitting for long periods of time. If the veins remain unsightly, painful or are still itching after the baby is born, you can have them removed, either by injection (sclerotherapy), in surgery (under general anaesthetic) or by laser (the procedure is called EVLT).

The pressure of your growing uterus on the veins in the pelvic region can also cause varicosities in the vulva or in your rectum in the form of haemorrhoids (see opposite).

HEARTBURN AND INDIGESTION

Heartburn (acid reflux) is very common in pregnancy, and almost every woman will experience it at some point. It can be horribly uncomfortable and I know women who have called the hospital thinking that something was severely wrong. For the absence of doubt, it is that burning sensation in your chest that you can occasionally feel all the way up into your throat. Some women say that they can even taste the acid at the back of the throat.

Reflux is a by-product of hormone production. Progesterone, which causes the muscles in your body to loosen, also causes a relaxation in the valve that links your stomach and your oesophagus, allowing acid from your stomach to seep upwards. As the baby gets bigger and the uterus pushes upwards, the burning sensation can be more severe and you may need to take liquid antacid to relieve it. Taller women don't appear to suffer as badly from indigestion, perhaps because there is more space for the baby. Women pregnant with twins, on the other hand, are more prone.

Amazingly, there is an upside to heartburn and the baby benefits from your

---

managing indigestion and heartburn

The following tips should help:

- ☉ avoid acidic foods (such as citrus juice), chocolate and very rich or spicy foods
- ☉ avoid alcohol and caffeinated drinks
- ☉ eat little and often
- ☉ try not to eat just before you go to bed – your body needs time to digest (two hours at least)
- ☉ prop yourself up on a pile of pillows when you go to sleep
- ☉ avoid restrictive clothing around the stomach area
- ☉ use a liquid antacid – the most common brand is Gaviscon
- ☉ in severe cases, your doctor may prescribe you Ranitadine tablets which inhibit acid production.

discomfort: the longer nutrients take to digest, the longer they remain in your bloodstream, which means the baby has longer to absorb them fully.

BACKACHE

One of the most common problems in pregnancy is backache. It can be caused by a number of factors, including the weight of your bump, the need to carry other children, bad posture (sometimes made worse by a heavier bust) and tension stored in the upper or lower back.

These factors are compounded by the pregnancy hormone progesterone which softens the ligaments, allowing the skeleton to expand and make room for the baby. It's worth getting into good habits now.

basic stretches for the back

There are a few basic stretches that can help you relieve tension in your back.

⊙ The first posture in this sequence is the cat stretch. Get down on all fours and arch your back like an angry cat. Try to feel each bone getting into the stretch and the gorgeous freedom of taking the weight off your lower back.

⊙ Feel the space in your middle back as the arch goes up and that sense of lightness in the stretch. Then dip your back the other way and raise your shoulders to feel the stretch in the other direction. Doing this a few times a week will greatly help relieve tension stored in the back area.

⊙ From all fours, sit your bottom onto the heels of your feet and tuck your knees underneath you. As your bump grows, you will need to make space for it so move your knees to a comfortable place either side of it.

⊙ Get comfortable and then lie forward with your face towards the floor and arms outstretched above you. It's a lovely stretch and you can feel the bones in your back enjoying it and a sense of release in your shoulders. Breathe into a stretch and enjoy the feeling for a few deep breaths. Your partner can also lay his hands on your lower back or sacrum area to help you relax, as suggested in the section on touch (see pages 73–4).

⊙ Come back up from that position and sit on your heels again. With your hands clasped, stretch your arms up above your head and turn your palms to the ceiling. Concentrate on looking forwards, keeping your chin down and your shoulders low. Try to extend that space between your shoulders and your ears.

PRACTISE GOOD POSTURE Bear in mind the following points:

- try not to slouch
- use the flat of your foot when you climb the stairs
- avoid 'bucket seats' (in which your bottom is lower than your knees) – these are bad for your back as well as for your circulation when you are pregnant
- always bend your knees and keep your back straight when lifting (although obviously it's not recommended for pregnant women to lift anything heavy). Also see the advice below on picking up toddlers
- avoid sitting in a 'reclining' position
- stand well – it may sound like the world's simplest advice, but it really makes a difference. Plant your feet firmly on the ground, pull your shoulders down and don't 'lock' your knees back.

PROTECT YOUR BACK WHEN PICKING UP TODDLERS Your back might be feeling a little creaky and it's important to know the correct way to lift a toddler when pregnant to avoid causing damage. A common complaint is back strain after putting a toddler in the car or buggy, or picking up a toddler by turning to the side while sitting or lying down. This kind of bending and twisting can be very bad for the back.

A demanding toddler might be particularly tricky to control, but you don't have any choice if you want to save yourself from back pain during the rest of your pregnancy. Get into the habit of picking up children only when absolutely necessary, (and only doing so with your knees bent and your back straight). I always encourage women to sit or crouch down first and then get their children to climb or jump onto their knee.

Childcare professionals advise that you don't blame the new baby for this change to the routine because it can cause

the wallaby stance

This standing position helps to take the weight off your back and make your pelvis feel 'free'. Imagine that you have a giant invisible tail, like a wallaby, that supports the base of your back. Stand with your feet flat on the ground and imagine them sinking into the earth and the imaginary tail holding you up. It's a relaxing pose if you're stuck in a queue in the supermarket or struck with pain while you're at work, or at the end of a hard day.

feelings of resentment in an older child. You can explain it by saying something like 'Mummy's back is a bit sore. Can you climb onto my lap for a hug instead of being picked up?' You can still give them plenty of affection, but try to save your poor back at the same time.

Toddlers and older children can also get into car seats by themselves, which can be a fun game, an example of how 'grown up' they are now, or may require every trick in the book – from distraction to bribery in the form of raisins, bananas, biscuits etc.

BUILD UP AN EXERCISE ROUTINE This should be gentle and regular. Osteopaths often see women who have done little exercise and are then surprised to find that their backs are not coping with the weight of the baby, especially in later weeks.

If you start now, a gentle but regular exercise routine will help strengthen your back enormously. Yoga stretches are also great for getting into areas of your spine that you wouldn't otherwise flex.

SWOLLEN LEGS (OEDEMA)

Swollen ankles are an almost universal symptom at some stage in pregnancy; you may notice a 'sock mark' on the ankles at the end of the day or, if you don't wear socks, a thickening in the area. As with varicose veins, this is in part caused by a slow down in your circulation causing your blood to pool and water to be forced down into the tissues around your ankles and feet. It's similar to the after-effects of a long-haul flight and is nothing to worry about.

Some women also notice their legs swelling, usually towards the end of the second trimester, and swelling in their

---

minimizing swelling

You can reduce swelling if you:

- ☉ get your feet above your heart – try lying on your back with your legs up against a wall (although this may become uncomfortable in the later stages of pregnancy)
- ☉ lie on your left-hand side with your right leg propped up on a small chair or on cushions
- ☉ prop your legs up on a stool while sitting down
- ☉ drink plenty of fluids – this prevents water retention
- ☉ avoid restrictive clothing
- ☉ use support tights – put them on first thing in the morning, before you get out of bed (make sure support tights are fitted properly; worn badly, support tights can make swelling worse)
- ☉ exercise – try a brisk walk or swim
- ☉ avoid too much salt in your diet.

hands (it's wise to remove rings from your fingers once this starts). While in the majority of cases there is nothing to worry about, do let your doctor or midwife know if you notice your face is starting to swell or that the swelling in your hands is severe. It can be a sign of pre-eclampsia, a serious and unpredictable condition that needs medical attention.

Unfortunately, some women are more prone to swelling in pregnancy, just as some women are naturally prone to fluid retention. The good news is that this is a short-lived symptom that will go after you have given birth.

ITCHY SKIN

Skin, because of hormonal changes, becomes drier during pregnancy and more likely to itch. In some cases you can actually see where your skin is stretching and, as it gets thinner, it is more sensitive to the clothes you are wearing – especially woolly jumpers, tights and socks in winter. Body temperature increases and some women sweat more during pregnancy, which can also irritate the skin. Itchiniess commonly occurs around the legs and bump, but also around the bottom.

A good moisturizer will help, and I suggest something unperfumed and very simple – expensive is not always better. You could try a gentle almond oil or olive oil, and it may also help to switch to a non-biological washing powder. Avoid having scratchy fabrics, such as wool, in direct contact with your tummy. Some women are so sensitive to itching, their skin is irritated even when they are wearing several soft layers underneath a jersey.

Itching can be a sign of obstetric cholestasis: if the palms or the soles of your feet are excessively itchy, and you feel you are scratching all the time – almost like a monkey – you need to see your doctor and have it checked out. (See page 328 for details of an obstetric cholestasis information organization.)

COLOSTRUM

Colostrum is the clear or slightly creamy liquid you will produce from your nipples in the first three to four days after birth, if you choose to breastfeed. It is very high in antibodies and helps build up your baby's immunity. It also has a mild laxative effect, which helps your newborn pass meconium – their first poo.

Many women start to leak colostrum during the second trimester, either in tiny amounts that are only noticeable if dried on your nipples, or in drops of liquid. This is completely normal. If you find the leaks excessive or embarrassing you can use breast pads to absorb it and prevent it showing in patches on your clothes. The fact that you are producing colostrum now will not affect your ability to breastfeed or the amount of milk you will produce after the baby is born.

STRETCH MARKS

Stretch marks, like morning sickness, are one of those extreme symptoms that give pregnancy a bad name. They are not universal, nor are they the end of the world. They can appear across the abdomen, on the thighs, the bottom or the breasts, and vary from pinkish lines to quite angry red 'scars'. As many as 75% of women experience stretch marks, although younger women, those with bigger babies or who are pregnant with twins, are more susceptible. You can be genetically predisposed to stretch marks and they may show more if you are fair or have red hair.

Even those who don't have them during pregnancy may find they suddenly appear a few days before giving birth. Like other untreatable pregnancy complaints it's best to deal with them by telling yourself that it's a small price to pay for a beautiful baby. Try not to obsess and remember – everyone experiences at least one bad pregnancy symptom.

There is little you can do to stop stretch marks, although a good diet and plenty of fluids may help. Oils and creams won't prevent them – it's the fibrous tissues beneath the skin that stretch – but a bump massage every evening is a gorgeous way to relax and helps you bond with your baby, your bump, and your partner if he wants to have a go.

Stretch marks don't completely disappear, but they do fade to silvery lines in time. I know women who proudly refer to stretch marks as their 'battle scars of pregnancy', others go for the gentler 'pregnancy lines'.

BABY KICKING

Feeling your baby's first kicks is a real milestone in pregnancy. It's one of those things in life you may have always wondered about – how it feels to have another being inside you. It's also a moment that helps you understand that your baby is a completely separate being – despite being entirely dependent on you. It's a really wonderful feeling.

Usually in a first pregnancy, kicking is felt by the mother from around 18–22 weeks, and this may be earlier with subsequent babies. The first few times you experience that bizarre little flutter, you may not be sure what it is. Some women describe it as a 'butterfly feeling' at the beginning of the second trimester, and first-time mothers are often not convinced of it until they feel a definite thump at around 18 to 23 weeks. Once you know the feeling, you don't forget it, which is partly why second time mothers often feel their babies kicking earlier. Slimmer women may also feel movement earlier.

As time goes on you will get to know your baby's routine. Some babies are prone to hiccups, which you can feel quite distinctly in the third trimester. You may find that the baby gets more active the moment you decide to rest – partly because your daytime rushing gently rocks the baby to sleep.

I think it's important to say here that some babies are more active than others – I had two kickers and two placid babies (and they are still the same today). It is important not to compare your baby's movements with those of its siblings or another pregnant woman's baby.

Although more an issue in the third trimester, if you do notice a distinct change in your baby's movements it's essential to see a midwife or obstetrician to check the baby is all right.

NOSEBLEEDS

Many women experience nosebleeds and bleeding gums when they are pregnant, and nosebleeds can be particularly bad when you have a cold. The pregnancy hormone progesterone is, once again, the culprit; it causes the soft mucous membranes to become more distended, making the capillaries weaker and more prone to bleeding.

If you feel the telltale 'fullness' of an oncoming nosebleed or a liquid sensation at the back of your throat, sit down. Pinch the softer area of your nose, just above your nostrils, for about 10 minutes.

The standard advice is to tip your head forward, allowing the blood to drain out rather than down the back of your throat. You need to keep pinching your nose for another 15 minutes or so to allow the blood to clot. You could also try a cold compress in the form of ice wrapped in a tea towel, which will help constrict the capillaries and reduce bleeding.

Try to blow your nose gently if you have a cold, and a soft or electric toothbrush will help with your gums. It's absolutely recommended that you see a dentist during pregnancy (see below).

PROBLEMS WITH TEETH AND GUMS

Many dentists subscribe to the adage 'a tooth per pregnancy'. Whether or not it is true that you lose a tooth every time you're pregnant, your baby is taking from you everything he or she needs, including calcium.

Most women experience some problem with their teeth and gums during pregnancy and many show some signs of 'pregnancy gingivitis', even if mild. The symptoms of gingivitis include swollen, tender and sensitive gums that are prone to bleeding, bad breath, or a funny taste in your mouth (which is different from the metallic taste of the first trimester). The best way to avoid gingivitis is by flossing, brushing regularly and keeping your mouth clean. You should see your dentist when you are pregnant. NHS dental treatment is free for pregnant women, so there is an incentive to go, especially if you haven't been for a while.

Women who are more exposed to stress and anxiety during pregnancy can start to grind their teeth in their sleep. For those who grind anyway, the habit can worsen. This can be another reason for teeth to crack or break, particularly in the vulnerable lower jaw. The first you may know about it is when your partner complains, but another telltale sign is jaw ache in the morning. Try breathing techniques before you go to sleep to relax your facial muscles and shoulders. In severe cases, you may need to use hot packs or flannels on your face to help relax the muscles.

SNORING AS A RESULT OF NASAL CONGESTION

Like teeth grinding, the first time you may learn of this is when your partner complains. In the same way that swollen nasal passages make pregnant women prone to nosebleeds and excess mucus, they can cause snoring. It's thought that as many as 23% of women start snoring for the first time during pregnancy, usually in the second trimester.

You can try to stop snoring by sleeping on your side (left-hand side is best), or by wearing nasal strips that you can buy at the chemist. The good news is that the pregnancy-related snoring, like so many other symptoms, disappears after the baby is born.

STRESS INCONTINENCE

Stress incontinence is what happens when you involuntarily lose urine while coughing, sneezing, exercising or lifting. It is extremely common, although not often discussed. In my experience, women are more likely to report it with second or subsequent pregnancies as a result of birth itself, but it happens to first time mothers when they are pregnant, too.

In pregnancy, there are a few causes of stress incontinence – the most basic of which is the pressure on your pelvic floor. It can be exacerbated by an untreated urinary tract infection and by constipation. A full bowel aggravates the problem. Like all pregnancy symptoms, you can be genetically pre-disposed to stress incontinence.

Birth itself is a common cause. Particularly at risk are those who experience a fast birth, a prolonged second stage, an assisted delivery (with forceps or ventous) or a very large baby. A distended (very full) bladder during labour can also cause stress incontinence, so make sure you go to the loo as often as possible (especially if you have an epidural); your birth partner can remind you.

If you are susceptible to stress incontinence, there are a few little tips that can help. Every time you feel you want to cough, pull up your pelvic floor (see pages 37–8), then cough. When you go to the loo, always check to see if you can squeeze any more out. It's important to make sure your bladder is completely emptied. This also prevents urinary infections. If you are waiting for the loo, a short-term solution is the old-fashioned, cross your legs and press the area to prevent a leak (although obviously this is not very dignified in public). You can also control the amount you drink before going about any activities where you may find you get caught short, such as a long walk, sex, a party or wedding with long queues for the loo, etc.

If you are finding stress incontinence embarrassing, there are pads you can buy from the chemist. I recommend that you use the pads specifically designed for stress incontinence.

If the problem is very severe after delivery, you may need to be referred to a physiotherapist who will help you redevelop your muscle strength in the area. They use a combination of exercises and 'vaginal cones', which teach you how to contract the muscles in the area. You can also be referred to an urogynaecologist who may recommend a course of drugs or injections to treat the problem. (See page 328 for contact details of a stress incontinence information service.)

VIVID DREAMS

It is completely normal to experience heightened colour in your dreams, as well as quite emotional dreams and classic 'anxiety' dreams, such as falling, being in an unfamiliar place or being 'out of control'. Women often dream about their unborn child – perhaps you will dream the sex of the baby or about the baby as a child or adult. You might even have quite disturbing dreams about your unborn child. For example I recently looked after a woman who dreamt she had given birth to a snake. She was worried about where in the house to put it and wasn't sure how to feed it. Another mother dreamt she'd had two small rabbits, another that her baby's tummy was made out of shark's teeth. These are normal manifestations of the anxiety you might be feeling about the arrival of the new baby and how you will cope.

You may also dream about people you haven't seen for a while or with whom you have unresolved issues. You may find yourself having highly erotic dreams and you may even orgasm in your sleep. This, too, is entirely normal.

INCREASED OR DECREASED INTEREST IN SEX

Many women report a huge interest in sex in the second trimester, in part because of the increase in energy, and also because their body is more engorged and orgasms are more powerful. You may have less of a desire for penetrative sex, but still crave a lot of physical affection. Many women want to be hugged much more than before. If this is the case, it may be that one solution is to enjoy foreplay with your partner and forsake penetrative sex for the time being.

Other women (particularly those who are uncomfortable with their changing body, or who are still feeling unwell) are not interested – and even put off by – the idea of sex. You may even shun physical intimacy with your partner entirely. All reactions are completely normal, in my experience, although any issues that are causing problems between you and your partner should be talked through.

sex is safe

Sex is completely safe in normal pregnancy and prior to birth. You cannot hurt the baby during lovemaking because the neck of the womb is closed by a thick mucous plug which protects the baby from infection. There are some circumstances when it is advisable to abstain from penetrative sex, such as if you have placenta praevia or vaginal bleeding. Oral sex (avoid your partner blowing air into the vagina), masturbation and the use of vibrators (provided they are clean) are all safe during pregnancy. If you have any concerns regarding sex during pregnancy, speak to your GP, obstetrician or midwife.

I don't believe women should ever feel pressurized into sex if they are not interested, and this can be particularly damaging to your relationship at a time when you are trying to forge intimacy, not resentment. It may be that intimacy takes on a different form in your relationship – perhaps you will talk more than before, perhaps you will spend more time doing things as a couple – such as going for walks, dinners, to the theatre or a museum.

Equally, if you have an increased libido and your partner is finding it difficult because of the presence of the bump, talk it through with him. Some men feel as if they are intruding on the baby's space, while others fear that they are going to 'poke the baby's eye out'. The baby will not be disturbed by your lovemaking – he or she is far away from the action, safely cushioned in the amniotic sac.

Your doctor or midwife will advise against penetrative sex if, for example, you have had a bleed, a cervical problem or a history of repeated miscarriage.

BRAXTON HICKS

Braxton Hicks, also referred to as practice contractions, occur when the uterus tightens and hardens in preparation for labour (see also pages 138–9). They usually begin at around 24–26 weeks, and should be painless, but you may notice your bump suddenly tightening and becoming almost rectangular in shape before returning to normal.

Late in pregnancy, some women report Braxton Hicks accompanied by backache and faint pains, which can be a sign that labour isn't too far away. If you have very strong and regular pain accompanying your uterus contracting, contact your hospital to rule out premature labour.

CRAMPS IN THE LEGS

Sudden, searing pain in your legs – sometimes in the middle of the night – is agony and can be terrifying, particularly for those who have never experienced it before.

Cramps can be caused by a number of different factors:

⊙ tired muscles – your entire system is overworked in pregnancy and muscles can seize up and cramp as a result. The area most likely to be affected is your calf muscle
⊙ the weight of the baby – this puts pressure on your circulation and in turn can cause cramps

- junk food – this is thought to contribute to leg cramps because of the high phosphorus content in processed foods
- mineral deficiencies – lack of salt, calcium, potassium, magnesium and Vitamin C could be to blame.

One way to avoid leg cramp is to do the exercise described on page 131. You should also practise 'airline exercises', such as rotating your ankle and flexing the calf muscle back and forth, before you go to bed.

If you experience a cramping episode, stretch your leg out and extend the heel hard, even if this hurts to begin with. The cramp should start to subside after a minute or so. Another way is to get your bare feet onto a cold floor, put your hands against the wall and stretch the area. (See also the advice on pages 131–2.) If you have consistent searing pain that is not relieved by stretching the muscles, you need to get help. Occasionally, pregnant women can develop a blood clot, which requires immediate medical attention.

SCIATICA

Sciatica is caused by the weight of your pregnancy putting pressure on the sciatic nerve. Generally you will feel it around your bottom, hips and thighs as a tingling or numbness, a little bit like pins and needles. If the pain appears to be travelling lower than your buttocks into your leg, report it to your doctor or midwife immediately. This can be more serious.

The best treatment for sciatica is to get blood circulating in the area. Try a hot compress or warm bath. Support the painful area with a pillow when you sleep.

your diet

As I mentioned before, you should really have a healthy eating plan in place by week 16. This means that you will have to jettison the easy sugary snacks of the first trimester and plan ahead for the moment hunger strikes.

A pain au chocolat may be what you want for breakfast, but chances are you'll be hungry again shortly afterwards. Foods that are immediately gratifying can put you into a cycle of a sugar high followed by a slump and encourage bad eating habits. A good tip for staving off hunger is to eat slow-burn carbohydrates in the morning, such as porridge, which you can jazz up nicely with sultanas, honey and/or banana. Many women swear by smoothies, although you need to watch your fruit intake over the whole day and keep your diet balanced.

snacks

Snacks mid-morning and mid-afternoon are a massive temptation when you are pregnant. Try to be disciplined and choose satisfying snacks that will stop you reaching for the biscuit jar or a pile of toast and jam. Try, for example:

- ⊙ oat cakes (plain, with goat's cheese, or mashed avocado)
- ⊙ rice cakes (a lighter, less filling, version of the above)
- ⊙ dried fruit (such as dates, prunes, apricots etc, which are all high in the right sugars, and also fibre)
- ⊙ yoghurt (go for something that doesn't have too much added sugar)
- ⊙ wholemeal bread (if you must head for the bread bin), with cheese, hoummous, mashed avocado or marmite, instead of jam
- ⊙ drinking more water (the more you drink the less likely you are to have swollen ankles too).

Obviously we can't always stay in control of our hunger pangs, so if you are craving chocolate and nothing I say is going to deter you, steer yourself towards black chocolate (70% cocoa plus), which is higher in iron and less sugary. It may be worth mentioning here that if you are still experiencing cravings for fatty or sugary foods, your body may not be getting all the nutrients it needs. If this is the case, you may need to take a vitamin supplement that is suitable for pregnant women.

ideas for fast, healthy meals

Many women are too tired to think about supper and just want to slump after a long day, either at work or with children. I encourage women to stock up a good store cupboard with things that can be prepared quickly. These include:

- brown pasta (or white, but brown is better for a pregnant system)
- brown or wild rice, lentils of any description (for example, Puy lentils can be knocked up in twenty minutes – eat with a fillet of grilled fish and some greens, or with a roasted chicken thigh and roasted vegetables, such as squash)
- couscous (again a quick option – you can use stock to give it more flavour and eat with, say, chicken and steamed vegetables)
- kidney beans (canned are good for a quick salad) or any other canned

---

on the run bag

I always suggest to the women I look after that they carry around in their bags an emergency supply of healthy snacks. One woman seemed to have an unending supply of nuts and raisins in her handbag. Here are some suggestions for your own 'on the run' bag:

- a bottle of water (you can fill this up whenever you pass a tap)
- raisins
- nuts and seeds
- an apple, banana or pear
- dried fruit – apricots, mango, figs and dates are good choices
- rice cakes
- sports bars (sample a variety first as some are horrible, and check the sugar content)
- (if you need sugar) squares of dark (70% plus) chocolate.

---

pulses that are quick to prepare, such as borlotti or flageolet beans (good with lamb)
⊙ chickpeas (used as per kidney beans, above)
⊙ canned tomatoes (along with an onion and a few herbs, cans of tomatoes are invaluable for a quick pasta, and you can add some steamed French beans or sautéed courgettes if you fancy something green).

You can also plan ahead by whipping up stews (meat or vegetable) and good soups and freezing them. If you don't find stew filling in itself, add some extra carbohydrate in the form of macaroni or pearl barley (follow the cooking instructions on the packet) or potatoes. There is also the good old-fashioned baked potato – although it does require cooking an hour and a half in advance if you don't have a microwave. I think good slow-burn evening meals help you feel energized the following day.

There are vegetables that help you to go to the loo and banish the cravings. These include:

⊙ squashes
⊙ jerusalem artichoke (great for a soup)
⊙ beetroot
⊙ spring or winter greens (these are cheap, incredibly nutritious and delicious stir-fried with garlic and a small amount of chilli)
⊙ sweet potato (like squash, you can roast sweet potato and eat it in a salad with, say, watercress and goat's cheese. Sprinkle a few pine nuts on top and you get the benefit of their nutritious oils, too
⊙ corn on the cob.

In summer, many of my mothers use filling salads to stave off the dreaded constipation. One favourite that has been passed around by mothers I have looked after is roasted beetroot and lentil salad with goat's cheese, figs and olive oil. Delicious, very nutritious and excellent for keeping constipation at bay.

You can jazz up many dishes with herbs – thyme is delicious with roasted vegetables, as is rosemary. Basil and parsley can be chopped into lentils and coriander is good with couscous. And it's especially important in summer to keep on drinking water.

I should add two more points about food and your growing baby. First, current thinking is that babies learn taste in the womb. They go on to enjoy different-flavoured food in breast milk. My colleague Michel Odent argues that a breast-fed baby is more adventurous with food later on in childhood than a formula-fed baby who doesn't experience the same variety of tastes.

My second point leads on from this. Learning to cook, or improving your skills, is something you will find invaluable when you have children. Even in the early days of weaning (when your baby is around five to six months old) the endless puréeing of carrots, sweet potatoes, broccoli etc, and batch freezing in advance, will be more manageable if you feel confident in the kitchen.

WEIGHT GAIN IN PREGNANCY

Putting on too much or too little weight in pregnancy is dangerous (see pages 64–5). Guidelines recommend that you put on just under half a kilo (1lb) per week in the second trimester, but my advice is that if you're weight was normal before you became pregnant, don't watch the scales.

Most women, however, are still concerned about the amount of weight they put on and often wonder what is normal. The range of 'normal' is fairly wide, but the average weight gain for a full-term pregnancy is 11kg (24.2lb).

That weight gain is broken down as follows:

Baby at birth	3.3kg (7.3lb)
Muscles in the uterus	900g (2lb)
Placenta	600g (1.3lb)
Extra weight in the breasts	400g (0.9lb)
Increase in blood volume	1.2kg (2.6lb)
Increase in fluid	2.6kg (5.7lb)

The issue of how you put on this weight in pregnancy is less straightforward. Some healthcare professionals argue that women don't need any extra calories in their diet for the first six months of pregnancy, and only about 200 extra calories per day during the last three months. Othes say that you should eat around 200 extra calories per day throughout pregnancy. Some say this should be 300 calories. (To give you an idea, 200 calories is two slices of toast, a jacket potato with 30g (1oz) of cheese or one slice of cheese on toast.)

One thing is for sure – do not allow someone else to dollop extra food onto your plate. The old 'eating for two' mentality has been universally abandoned.

feeling confident during pregnancy

Many women battle with their appearance. I always assure them that it is a state of mind. Pregnant women are beautiful. However, some women see their bump as part of the celebration of pregnancy – they wear tight clothes to show it off and feel and look great – while others do their best to hide their bump, perhaps believing that they look 'fat', or just not wanting to draw attention to it to avoid being touched, commented on and thus feeling like public property.

getting your wardrobe right

The key has to be finding the balance between being comfy and feeling confident. You can learn to adapt outfits. For example, if you have oversized shirts, try using a loose belt beneath your bump to show where the bump ends and you begin. It may make you feel less like you are wearing a tent. Dresses or tops that tie underneath the bust have the same effect – you can find good maternity wrap dresses quite cheaply and they have the advantage of growing with you as you get bigger. One tip from a mother I know: if you increase the size of your jewellery, it can have the effect of making you smaller.

Another tip is that, if you are very conscious of varicose veins, wear leggings underneath dresses to conceal them. Tracksuit bottoms – make sure they have a wide elasticated waist so that they don't fall down the whole time – are a great pregnancy wardrobe staple. Many women live in them in the later weeks.

Shoes are important – your feet need to be comfortable, they are supporting all that extra weight in pregnancy. If you can't bear a Birkenstock sandal, try a good brand of trainers or, if you need something smarter, a supported flat shoe, such as a loafer. Sarah Jessica Parker may well have worn them to great effect on the red carpet while pregnant, but I'm afraid high heels are a no-no in pregnancy. They place huge strain on your back and are bad for your feet.

comments about your bump

Pregnant women are often approached and touched by strangers, which can be unpleasant. Some compare it to being assulted. Another hazard is the comments from those around you – friends or even strangers. For some bizarre reason, people think they have a licence to comment on the size of a pregnant woman. It's ludicrous when you think about it; such open comments would be considered rude in any other context.

Among the more ridiculous comments, which most women hear at least once in pregnancy, are:

- ☉ 'You're massive! Are you overdue?'
- ☉ 'Can't be long now. You're only five months? Really?'
- ☉ 'You're going to have that baby any minute!'
- ☉ 'Are you sure there aren't twins in there?'
- ☉ 'Don't have that baby here!'

Even other mothers, who should know better, occasionally join in:

- ☉ 'Gosh, I didn't show until way later than you.'
- ☉ 'Wow, you're big for four months.'

You'll need every ounce of my mantra 'patience, patience' not to react or feel hurt by other people's comments, but it can help to know that the vast majority of people don't know what they are talking about when it comes to bump size.

I looked after one woman with a bump size that was bang-on average, who laughingly told me how one day a woman had been shrieking at her for being 'far too small for your dates' and asked her, 'Are you eating properly?' Not one hour later, someone else randomly commented, 'Wow, you're really quite big, aren't you?' She merely rolled her eyes and got on with her day.

preparing your body for birth

The best thing you can do to increase your chances of a relatively easy, safe and (if you wish) natural birth is to exercise regularly during pregnancy. Labour is a marathon. Physical fitness and stamina will give you a head start.

The majority of women in this trimester have increased energy so, if you haven't already, start thinking about a gentle exercise routine. This can be as simple as a stroll around the park, or as energetic as a 20-minute swim three mornings a week – although obviously don't overdo it, and build up any exercise you do slowly and gently. It's important that you don't push yourself too hard. You should stop at once if you feel any pain at all, feel dizzy, nauseous or faint, or if you experience any shortness of breath. If you decide to practise at home, remember to avoid lying flat on your back for extended periods of time beyond your second trimester. Consult your GP before embarking on any new or vigorous exercise programme.

There are good reasons for doing exercise now: as well as preparing you for the 'marathon of labour', it improves circulation, keeps haemorrhoids at bay, promotes feel-good hormones (endorphins) and encourages you to feel more positive about yourself, your body and your birth.

yoga

Women who do pregnancy yoga with a good, experienced teacher tend to do very well in labour. This is partly because of the concentration on breathing techniques, but also because they have increased flexibility and practise positions that are exceptionally useful during labour. I've found those women who have done a class a week of yoga tend to come into hospital later in labour, are more confident about childbirth and feel stronger after birth.

Yoga stretches also help with some of the fundamental problems of pregnancy, such as bad posture, backache and poor circulation (which can cause problems such as varicose veins). Another benefit of a regular class is the opportunity to shut out the rest of the world completely for a while and exist in a totally calm and relaxed space. It is great to be able to draw on that experience – and withdraw to that place – during labour.

My own take on yoga is that it is invaluable during pregnancy, especially if you want a natural birth. The spiritual aspect of yoga is, I think, particularly good for training you to adjust mentally to focusing in on your body. If you practise yoga enough, this will become an almost unconscious reaction to labour.

Even if you can only afford a couple of classes, it's a worthwhile investment. You can follow it up in your own time when you are confident you know the positions and will not cause yourself any injury.

yoga for pregnancy and birth

A word on yoga from my colleague Fenella Lindsell of YogaBugs Ltd:

'Labour is probably one of the most physical things you'll ever do, so preparation for it is very important! Yoga empowers women to believe in the strength of their bodies and the focus of their minds. Birth is such a natural process and yoga helps to facilitate this natural journey to life. It is important that if you are starting yoga that you first consult your medical practitioner and that you work with a qualified ante natal yoga teacher. Ideally it is best to start yoga after 14 weeks, when the pregnancy is well established.

The breathing exercises help to calm the body and focus the mind whilst creating an important connection between mother and baby. Learning to breathe correctly is invaluable during labour for pain relief and to help women to stay focused on the contractions.

Posture work helps to build strength, endurance and improve circulation. At the same time some of the sequences can help to generate courage and improve self-confidence. Equally, postures can be helpful to turn breach babies, improve digestion and enable women to relax more easily.

Relaxation, visualisation and meditation techniques help women to find the stillness they need to connect with their babies. In today's busy world, women find it increasingly difficult to find time to get to know their baby and see life as starting when their new baby arrives. Creating time for togetherness after the physical practise of yoga can help to build a strong union between mother and baby which will continue throughout their lives ahead.'

(See page 328 for contact details for YogaBugs.)

the gym

If you go to the gym, a gentle workout can be highly beneficial during pregnancy. If you are not used to the gym, start off with some gentle walks on the treadmill. You can increase your pace and the amount of time you spend doing it in time. It may be worth getting an instructor to guide you to the machines that are best during pregnancy. Many women, however, like the cross-trainer (which can help you build up mental stamina) and to cycle.

I am a gym, swim and cycling fan, but came to exercise late in life, in my 40s. With an instructor, Alecia Van Wyke, I have learned to retrain my core muscles. Alecia recommends aqua aerobics and swimming for pregnancy and says that they not only improve your stamina but also lift your mood considerably. She says that the most significant changes to take place in a pregnant woman's body are cardiovascular. Your body's blood volume increases by 40%, and the heart has to work harder to circulate it, increasing heart rate and cardiac output.

Her advice is to watch your heart rate and try to ensure it doesn't increase over 140 beats per minute (bpm) for longer than one minute as this can result in increased cardiac output. She also advises that while exercising, you keep your body temperature down (hence, don't use the steam room), exercise in short bursts, avoid lying on your front to exercise and avoid excessive physical or mental pressure.

caution

If you experience any of the following you need to stop exercising immediately and contact your GP:

- ⊙ vaginal bleeding
- ⊙ loss of amniotic fluid
- ⊙ dizziness
- ⊙ fainting
- ⊙ nausea or vomiting
- ⊙ oedema (swelling)
- ⊙ a reduction in the amount the baby moves
- ⊙ high blood pressure
- ⊙ pre-eclampsia
- ⊙ pregnancy induced hypertension.

pilates

Many of the women I look after also swear by pregnancy Pilates. This form of exercise concentrates on working the muscles that are used for movement and posture, in order to build strength, flexibility and coordination. You can work at a slow pace or in a more 'dynamic' way. Most pregnancy Pilates is done on mats, but if you are experienced you may also be using specialized equipment.

The 'core muscles' that are central to the practice are put under a lot of strain in pregnancy. Regular Pilates sessions with an instructor qualified to help pregnant women will therefore be hugely beneficial. Like yoga, Pilates also places great emphasis on improving breathing techniques that can also be useful for labour. It also places emphasis on that all important pelvic floor. One function of the pelvic floor muscles (to contract and to hold) can be trained with Pilates-based exercises where the focus is on 'lifting' the pelvic floor and sustaining the engagement while moving. For many women this helps with pelvic stability and other issues such as incontinence. (See page 329 for how to find classes near you.)

swimming

Swimming is a lovely exercise for pregnant women because the water creates a natural support for your bump. Technically you can swim anytime in pregnancy and from the sixth week after birth.

If you are just beginning an exercise routine now, it may be the first time in a while that you have felt so supported and your baby can probably feel this extraordinary freedom too. Swimming exercises the body in a gentle way, without the high-impact of running or the gym. Less stress is placed on the joints and the cool water prevents the body heating up too much.

Even walking in water can help build up the body's muscles and stamina and improve circulation, so it's a good way to start if you are building up your exercise routine gradually.

If you use breaststroke, you can build up a gentle rhythm as well as thinking about your breath with each sweep of your arms. I often encourage women to do what I call 'breaststroke breathing' during labour, so it's helpful to get really familiar with this exercise and the kind of breath you are using.

I should add a word of caution, however: if you have been experiencing severe back pain, or you are using swimming to build up the muscles in your back, it is recommended that you use backstroke rather than breaststroke, which can exacerbate severe back pain.

getting baby into the best position for birth

Towards the end of the second trimester your baby will begin to settle into position, and you can influence your labour by taking steps to ensure 'optimal foetal positioning'.

The best position for a baby to be in for birth is occipito anterior (see below, first diagram) – the baby's head is down and facing your spine, their chin tucked on their chest and their legs and arms are crossed. A baby who begins labour in this position has a better chance of a straightforward birth.

A baby whose position is occipito posterior (see below, second diagram) – when the baby faces your abdomen and your spines are parallel – is more likely to have problems progressing in labour. Similarly, babies born 'face first', instead of with their chins tucked under, are likely to have longer labours.

If your baby is diagnosed as being occipito transverse (see below, third diagram), then their back is facing towards your side. In most cases a baby that is occipito transverse will usually turn occipito anterior during labour.

Finally, you may find that your baby is breech (see below, fourth diagram). Only 2.5% of babies are breech presentation and around 90% of those are now delivered by Caesarean section, especially if it is a first birth. You can deliver a breech baby naturally, although this comes with some risks that need to be thought through carefully. I recommend you have all the information at your fingertips and discuss it with both your midwife and partner. See pages 161–7 for more information on breech babies.

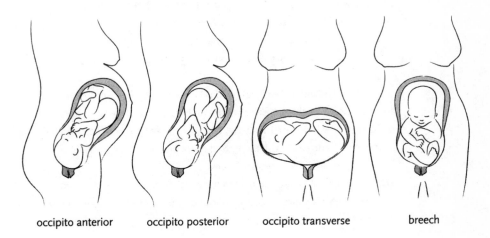

occipito anterior   occipito posterior   occipito transverse   breech

INFLUENCING YOUR BABY'S POSITION

There are a few factors that can contribute to the baby settling into a good position. Practising good posture such as walking with a straight back and relaxed shoulders, and finding ways of giving your pelvis 'freedom' both help. Below are some tips for getting your baby into a good position for birth.

USE A BIRTHING BALL It may sound ridiculous, but using a birthing ball (or a gym or exercise ball) as a chair at your desk, particularly if you spend long hours in front of a computer, is good not just for your back, but for the baby's position and for your posture. (See page 329 for sources of birthing balls.)

TURN YOUR CHAIR AROUND AND KNEEL ON IT If you can't use a birthing ball, you can adapt your existing situation. For example, you can turn the chair around so that the back of the chair faces your desk and kneel on the seat for a few minutes everyday. This position automatically gives your spine and pelvis freedom and helps the baby achieve a better position.

AVOID 'COMFY' SOFAS, BUCKET SEATS OR SITTING TOO LONG IN ONE POSITION Soft chairs, armchairs and sofas may look very enticing, but they can be terrible for posture, as can sitting in one place for too long. If there is no other option, chose the floor over a 'comfy' sofa – you can sit with your back straight, or with your tail bone propped up with a thin cushion.

GET DOWN ON ALL FOURS If you are forced to sit in one position all day, you need to give your back and pelvis a well-deserved rest. One way of doing this is to get onto all fours and swinging your hips in a figure-of-eight shape, which is a good way to release tension in the area.

LIE ON YOUR LEFT SIDE WHILE YOU SLEEP Whenever possible, and especially at night, get into the habit of lying on your left-hand side with a cushion between your knees. If you think it will make you more comfortable in the position, prop your right leg up on a stack of cushions or a child's chair.

LIE ON YOUR BACK FOR A FEW MINUTES EACH DAY While you still can, you may find it nice to lie flat on your back for a few minutes each day. This is great for relaxing the spine, which is working hard during pregnancy.

reducing stress

While there is no solid medical evidence that emotional stress can cause miscarriage or premature birth (indeed one study has shown that women in war zones tend to deliver later), some obstetricians believe stress can contribute to complications, including intrauterine growth restriction. Other studies suggest that high levels of stress hormones can cross the placenta and affect the baby into childhood. The effect of prenatal stress certainly warrants more research.

On a more straightforward level it is easy to see how stress can affect your pregnancy. If you have disrupted sleep, develop bad eating habits, or stress is making you feel frustrated, angry and isolated, it will have a negative impact on your pregnancy.

If you are doing a lot of physical work, you need to ensure you are taking care of yourself and not doing any more than you can manage or becoming overtired or weak from work. Too much physical stress – unlike emotional stress – can bring on preterm labour.

My view is that stress in normal life is not good, so stress when you are pregnant is doubly unwelcome. The best way to approach stress, as with all problems that seem overwhelming, is to take each 'stressful' issue and deal with them one at a time.

Another way to counteract stress is to look for balances in your life. An hour of yoga or the gym, for example, may counteract a whole day of pressure at work. Equally, a walk in the park or coffee with a friend might put you in a different frame of mind.

WORK

If your work is excessively stressful (either because you work very long hours, because you travel all the time, or because of the kind of material that you deal with) and causes you anxiety, you need to take a step back. Pregnancy is your priority right now. Can you cut your hours back? Get someone to share your workload? Perhaps you can cut back on travel or work from home occasionally. Ask if you can be exempt from dealing with certain situations or 'cases' if, say, they are distressing.

preparing for parenthood

Now is a good time for making practical preparations for your baby's arrival. This is the time to make the announcement at work that you are pregnant, and to start planning for your maternity leave. And with the morning sickness and overwhelming tiredness behind you, the reality of having a baby may be very exciting right now, so buying the essentials you'll need to look after your baby is not only practical but can be a lot of fun.

telling your colleagues

If you haven't already, now is the time to tell your boss that you are pregnant (or, if you are the boss, to tell your employees). Practical decisions about your role need to be considered. These may be decisions made by you, they may be made by your employer. For example, who will do your work when you are away? What needs to be handed over? What needs to be completed in advance of your maternity leave?

making changes at work

It is important to address your day-to-day working practices and whether they are appropriate now that you are pregnant. Remember – don't be shy. You have rights at work and your priority has to be your pregnancy. If you work in a big office, for example, the Occupational Health department may want to chat to you about your duties. If you work late shifts, can you switch? Can you have more breaks in the day to move around? How easy is it for you to move around? Are the conditions you work in comfortable? They may also want to look at your work station. For example:

- is your computer at a good height?
- is your chair comfortable (as I've said before, anything resembling a bucket seat is not good for your back or pelvis)?
- is there a footstool available?

Obviously if you are very close to some of your work colleagues, they may already know your exciting news. However, it always makes things easier if your boss hears your news from you, rather than on the grapevine. Even if you are bursting with excitement, try to keep a professional lid on it. Make an appointment to see your boss and tell them in private.

Bosses don't always react in the way we would like them to and you shouldn't let this affect you. Their job is merely to work out how your news will affect their business, so don't let a blaze or brusque reaction put a dampener on your happy announcement. I've heard of many bosses who have been delighted for their employees. I've also heard a few horror stories, including the mother-to-be who was asked, 'Who is the father? I wasn't aware you even had a boyfriend.'

your maternity leave

Most women chose to start their maternity leave between 34 and 36 weeks, however you are legally allowed to start it anytime after 28 weeks. The question of whether you should work right up until your due date is a difficult one, especially if you are self-employed. You have to decide depending on how you feel and how physically or emotionally demanding you are finding your work.

I hear that there is something of a fashion for some high-powered women to 'play chicken' with their due date, and this is born more out of competitive work environments and midwives than the interests and wishes of the mother. Many obstetricians will encourage women to have some time off before a first birth to acclimatize to their changing situation. It's good to have some time to focus totally on the event ahead and to properly relax, without distraction. (See page 328 for details of services that supply information about employment and your rights.)

buying essentials for your baby

It's typically suggested that you should think about buying the essentials for the nursery at anytime from 26 weeks onwards. I think this is good advice as some items, such as cots, can have long delivery times.

Excited first-time parents often buy far more than they need – especially when

the basic essentials

CLOTHES

⊙ VESTS

These are little body suits either with no arms, short sleeves or long sleeves with poppers that do up between the legs (to make nappy access easy). In high summer they can sleep in just a vest, in winter they can wear a vest underneath a sleep suit.

⊙ SLEEP SUITS

These are sometimes called 'baby gros' and are the all-in-one long-sleeved outfits that have poppers running all the way down the front and on the inside of both legs. Winter versions have feet, summer versions may not. You can buy newborn sleep suits that have a flap of extra material to pull over your baby's hands to stop them scratching themselves. Alternatively you can buy scratch mitts.

⊙ HAT

This is an essential in winter. Body heat can escape from your head and newborns' heads are large compared to their bodies. The pure cotton hats are less scratchy and can be worn under something warmer if you need to be outside and it's very cold.

⊙ SCRATCH MITTS

Newborns can have long nails, which are difficult to cut. Because they have little control over their little hands, babies are prone to scratching their own faces, which hurts.

⊙ KNITTED BOOTIES (in winter)

⊙ WOOLLEN CARDIGAN (in winter)

⊙ WOOLLEN BLANKET (in winter)

Do keep blankets away from the baby's face.

⊙ SNOWSUIT (in winter)

Be sure to remove the snowsuit once you are back inside. Newborns find it hard to regulate their temperature and can overheat.

⊙ WOOLLEN MITTENS (in winter)

SLEEP ACCESSORIES

⊙ SWADDLING BLANKET

The T-shirt material versions are best because they are stretchy, but some women prefer using a holey blanket.

⊙ MOSES BASKET AND STAND

Babies can sleep in this basket until around eight to twelve weeks.

⊙ SHEETS FOR THE MOSES BASKET

⊙ COT

⊙ COT SHEETS

⊙ COT BLANKET

The ones with holes (cellular blankets) are recommended in case the blanket rides up to the baby's face. These can also be used for swaddling.

⊙ BABY MONITOR

CLEAN UP AND GROOMING

⊙ MUSLIN SQUARES

You may never have heard of muslins before, but you will never forget them once you have a newborn. They are essential for mopping up everything, from 'spit up' (regurgitated milk) to wee during a changing session. You will learn to wear one over your shoulder at all times – and they can even be used as an impromptu nappy for little boys!

⊙ NAPPY CHANGE MAT
⊙ NAPPIES
Disposable or washable, but if washable, you may also need Napisan.
⊙ COTTON WOOL BALLS
For wiping the baby's bottom – baby wipes are often said to be too harsh for newborn skin.
⊙ NAPPY RASH CREAM
⊙ BABY MASSAGE OIL
Use something that is recommended for newborns to avoid a skin reaction. Pure almond oil is good; you can also use olive oil.
⊙ SOFT SPONGE
For washing in the bath.
⊙ BABY TOWELS
You can buy ones with a hood.
⊙ FLANNEL
⊙ THERMOMETERS
One for your baby's bath and bedroom, another to check his or her temperature.
⊙ NAIL CLIPPERS
See note on scratch mitts above.
⊙ SOFT HAIRBRUSH

OTHER EQUIPMENT
⊙ BOUNCY CHAIR
For sitting the baby in.
⊙ PLAY MAT
Sometimes called a 'baby gym'. This is a soft and colourful mat with an arched arm on which you can attach dangling toys for the baby to play with.
⊙ PRAM/PUSHCHAIR
If you are buying a pushchair, check it reclines flat and is therefore suitable for newborns. Those that don't recline are only recommended for babies over three months.
⊙ PRAM/PUSHCHAIR PARASOL (in summer)
⊙ SLING
To carry the baby in – useful when you need to be 'hands-free'.
⊙ REAR FACING CAR SEAT
Get one even if you don't have a car (be very careful if you buy a car seat second-hand – see cautions on page 110)

FEEDING
If you want to express breast milk (so that someone else can feed the baby from a bottle), or use formula milk, you will also need:
⊙ STERILIZING UNIT/ EQUIPMENT
⊙ BOTTLES
⊙ TEATS
⊙ EXPRESSING MACHINE
⊙ FREEZER BAGS FOR BREAST MILK

it comes to clothes, which babies grow out of with remarkable speed – if they ever fitted into them. For example, you may buy 'newborn' size sleep suits, only to discover that your whopping bundle of joy has skipped the first size of sleep suit completely and has moved straight into the '0–3 months' size. For this reason, avoid the temptation to unpack everything as soon as you have bought it – it may need to be returned.

SECOND-HAND EQUIPMENT

Why not? There is nothing wrong with a good old-fashioned hand-me-down, as long as it is in reasonable condition. You are going to spend a small fortune on your offspring as life goes on, so you may as well start thinking on a budget now. You can acquire good-quality second-hand equipment from a variety of sources – friends and family, the internet (try parenting forums and ebay), jumble sales, charity shops and NCT second-hand sales.

CAUTIONS Obviously you always need to be careful when buying things second-hand.

- ⊙ Car seats: Do not buy second-hand car seats unless you are absolutely sure you know its entire history. A car seat can be dangerously flawed if it has been in a car accident, even if there are no visible signs of damage.
- ⊙ Pushchairs: Check that a second-hand pushchair complies with British Standard BS 7409. You also need to check the brakes work and that there are no sharp points jutting out.
- ⊙ Mattresses: Most companies recommend that you buy new cot and Moses basket mattresses for each new baby.
- ⊙ Clothes: Wash in non-biological powder before use.
- ⊙ Teats and dummies: Don't use second-hand teats or dummies.
- ⊙ Electrical goods: Make sure these have been tested by someone who knows what they are doing before you use them in the baby's nursery.
- ⊙ Toys: You can check online for information on toys recalled by the manufacturers for any reason.

becoming a father

The second trimester can be a puzzling time for Dads – their partner has changed from the always exhausted, faintly (or horribly) nauseous, highly strung individual they supported through the first trimester, into an extraordinary superwoman, with huge energy reserves and an abundance of patience and good will. Or has she?

In truth, her hormones may still be raging in the background and, unfortunately, a pregnant woman is still an unpredictable woman. Dads still need to walk the journey with their pregnant partners and be as supportive as possible. Most importantly, they need to be ready to talk through the difficult issues you are both facing in the coming weeks.

Bottling things up doesn't help. When I do my Birth Rehearsal (see pages 175–7), I address it to both men and women and often find that men have a surprising amount to say. The floodgates open once they realize there are other men in a similar situation, facing similar challenges. You both need to be as candid as possible with each other – becoming a family is a wonderful journey but it can also be difficult.

COMMON CONCERNS FROM DADS

'IT'S AS IF THE BABY HAS COME BETWEEN US ALREADY' Dads often feel that the changes in their partner's body correspond with a growing distance in the relationship. I tell them to try to see things from the mother's perspective – she is facing a dramatic change in body image and may not be feeling herself.

The baby is getting bigger, becoming harder to ignore. It's harder for the mother-to-be to sleep and life is getting a little less comfortable generally. I ask fathers to think about the way they treat her during this time.

Being supportive of each other, both in practical ways and with affection may help both of you bridge any gaps that you are concerned about.

'I FEEL TORN BETWEEN MY WIFE AND MY MOTHER' Grandparents often feel they have a lot of advice to give their children when they become parents for the first time. Some of it is wonderfully helpful; some is not. Things change a lot in one generation. The problem of interfering grandparents is almost as common as morning sickness. It's important to set boundaries now.

Dads often say that they find it hard to negotiate between the two strong women in their lives. I usually advise them to prioritize: your partner and your baby need you right now. Dads can give their own mothers a role in the baby's future that will allow them to be involved but not to interfere too much.

Sensitive situations need to be dealt with carefully, but also firmly. Grandparents are an amazing layer in your new family and you need to work out a way of embracing them in a way that works for everyone.

'WHY IS SHE SO SENSITIVE?' One of the oldest complaints in the book is that Dads make the most extraordinarily insensitive comments. My general advice to Dad is to listen to her. Don't comment on her size or shape, and don't underestimate how tired she is feeling. A pregnant mother needs the emotional equivalent of having her pillows fluffed regularly. That need becomes doubly important once the baby arrives, sleep patterns are all over the place and tempers are frayed.

THINKING AHEAD TO AFTER THE BIRTH

I always tell Dads to look after the new mum – she is looking after your baby. Both mother and father have needs after the baby is born, but it's worth flagging up things that you may be concerned about now. Think through the possible sticking points. For example:

DOES DAD'S JOB MEAN HE NEEDS AN UNINTERRUPTED NIGHT'S SLEEP? If so, you may need to work out sleeping arrangements now. Can Dad sleep in the spare room or on the sofa in the early weeks? Can Mum sleep in the baby's room? What works for both of you?

DOES DAD EXPECT A TIDY HOUSE AND FOOD ON THE TABLE WHEN HE GETS HOME FROM WORK? The arrival of a new baby can turn a perfectly tidy house with a well-stocked fridge into a famine-stricken bombsite. Brace yourselves now. Is an immaculate house and plenty of food important? If so, you may need to organize extra help. If you expect food to be ready when you get home, you may need to stock up your freezer with pre-prepared food that you can both live on in the early weeks.

HOW IMPORTANT IS IT FOR DAD TO 'WET THE BABY'S HEAD'?
Wetting the baby's head is the old-fashioned idea of celebrating the new arrival with several large drinks while the new mother is still in hospital (or tended to by family). Be sure, however, that the new mother is not left alone for too long, or at least has someone to call if she needs anything/in an emergency.

A word of caution too: don't sleep with the baby in the bed if either parent has been drinking.

HOW IMPORTANT IS IT FOR DAD TO MAINTAIN A SOCIAL LIFE
ONCE THE BABY ARRIVES? A new mother needs as much support as possible in the early weeks. Organize a balance between the needs of mother and baby and the needs of Dad. Can he be back at a set time? Can he have a set role – say the 10 or 11 o'clock feed (if you have one)?

your developing baby

The moment you both feel the baby kick is almost the first moment you can really imagine the three (or more) of you as a family. The second trimester is the most extraordinarily wonderful stage for most mothers, but it's also a time that allows your partner to step into their role more consciously.

Your baby is developing at an extraordinary rate and, at around 15 weeks he can hear your heartbeat, your voice and the lower register in your partner's voice. Through sound, and the familiarity of your touch, he starts to get to know you. As the trimester goes on, he will become much more active and, by the end of this period, you will really start to feel as if you are getting to know him.

weeks 13–17: time for expansion

You may now be able to hear your baby's heartbeat on your midwife's hand-held Doppler device placed on your tummy, but don't worry if you can't; some babies' heartbeats aren't detected until 18 weeks. Inside, your baby's body is now covered in fine hair called lanugo that will continue to grow until around 26 weeks. Her bones are getting stronger and, as her body grows, she takes on a more recognizable baby shape. Her fingernails are fully formed and she may even start to suck her thumb.

Your baby's chest might rise and fall in preparation for breathing, although the lungs are not fully formed until around 37 weeks, when the likelihood of your baby being born with breathing difficulties is 1%. By this time she may even be coughing and hiccupping.

Your baby's hearing and taste buds are developing and some doctors believe that the baby can taste elements of the food you are eating. A white waxy substance called vernix covers the baby's skin to protect it from drying out while in the amniotic fluid.

By now, your baby is in constant motion, touching her face, holding on to the umbilical cord, her feet touching the walls of the womb. Around this time you may well feel some little flutters – the first feelings of a life within. I remember these seeming like soft butterfly kisses. Over the next few weeks these feelings will become more profound.

As your womb stretches like a balloon to accommodate your baby, she grows bigger, and so does the placenta, the umbilical cord and the amniotic sac. You will notice this growth by watching the ever-increasing size of your abdomen.

weeks 18–23: a perfect miniature person

By 18–20 weeks, your baby is a perfect person in miniature. He can pull a whole range of facial expressions, most of them involuntary reflexes, including smiling, frowning and even 'crying'. Your baby can hear your heartbeat, the swishing sound of your blood moving through your arteries and veins, and the muffled sound of your voice and your partner's voice. He can also hear music, as well as loud noises that may startle him.

By 20 weeks your baby has completed half of his journey into the world and you are half way through your pregnancy. He has hair (lanugo) over his face and body, his arms and legs are very skinny as there is no fat on them yet, and his head makes up one-third of his entire length. At your 20-week scan, you will be able to determine your baby's sex (if you want to find out). The ultrasonographer can show you all the different parts of your baby on the screen – the little head, stomach bubble, face, spine, brain, heart, bladder and limbs. The vocal cords can be viewed as well and, if they are moving a lot, perhaps your baby will be a chatterbox later on!

Your baby's reproductive organs are continuing to form. Baby girls have around six million eggs at around this time. Amazingly this figure will diminish to around one million by birth.

By 24 weeks, your little baby has crossed the viability line, which means that, if he were born he would have a fighting chance of survival.

weeks 24–27: starting to feel the squeeze

By 24 weeks your baby's vital organs are becoming increasingly sophisticated and she has taken on the appearance of a newborn, although she still needs to fatten up as she only weighs as much as a bag of sugar – about 500g – and is about 24cm long. If you are expecting twins, they may already be 'playing' – touching and kicking each other.

The baby now recognizes your voice and responds to it and may also kick in response to a gentle pressing of your tummy. If your partner cups his hands over your bump and speaks to the baby, he will probably get a kick or a nudge from inside. This is a great way for your partner to begin a physical bond with her.

At 26 weeks, your baby is in full growth-spurt mode and is now approximately 32cm long and weighs about 900g. She occupies a lot more of the womb space and her legs are now curled up due to limited space. She spends longer periods sleeping. She can now open her eyes, and her brain is constantly developing.

By now you may have become attuned to your baby's sleeping and waking routine. This routine may form the pattern of your baby's sleeping and waking times when she initially arrives, although she will quickly adapt to any routine you put her in once she is in your care on the outside.

your antenatal care

You will see your GP, midwife or obstetrician (depending on what kind of care you are having) more frequently in the second trimester. You can expect to have a check-up at around 16–18 weeks, then another to correspond with your 20–22-week scan. Thereafter, you will be seen every three weeks during this trimester.

antenatal appointments

Your GP, midwife or obstetrician will routinely check the following:

- your urine
- your blood pressure
- the measurement of your uterus (it should correspond approximately in centimetres to the number of weeks you are)
- the position (presentation) of your baby
- the foetal heartbeat (although you may not be able to hear it until 18 weeks) using a hand-held machine called a Doppler ultrasound device or a Pinard stethoscope
- the lie of your baby
- for swelling in the face, hands and feet
- in some cases you will also be weighed (although I don't generally do this, unless I think there is a cause for concern).

Obviously the frequency with which you see your caregivers will also depend on whether you are 'high risk' or 'low risk' and whether you are expecting more than one baby. Most women who are being treated on the NHS and have low risk pregnancies will not be scanned after 20–22 weeks if everything is normal.

YOUR OBSTETRIC NOTES
It is now universally recommended that women carry their maternity notes with them at all times. This is particularly important if you are travelling abroad, although you may be given an abbreviated record with brief notes.
Obviously it's important that you keep these notes safe. There are several

reasons why you carry them.

- ⊙ You are in charge of your own journey through pregnancy. You need to show these notes whenever you are seen by a GP, midwife, obstetrician or doctor.
- ⊙ It gives any medical personnel that you need to see, for whatever reason, a detailed description of how your pregnancy is progressing.
- ⊙ If you need treatment in an emergency and you cannot speak for yourself, your notes can speak for you.

HOW TO READ YOUR OBSTETRIC NOTES Here I will run through everything you are likely to see in your notes. Don't worry too much if there are things I describe here that aren't on your records – hospitals differ in what they include. If you have any concerns, you can always ask your GP or midwife. Your notes are technically the property of the NHS – or your private clinic – and they carry the name of your hospital, your hospital number and a list of telephone numbers for emergencies.

Your obstetric notes are a record of your current pregnancy, past pregnancies and the outcomes, any existing medical conditions, allergies or any prescribed medicine you are taking. They also chart your progress through your current pregnancy from an emotional and physical as well as medical perspective. They include details of your baby, the date of your LMP (last menstrual period), your EDD (estimated due date) and results of any ultrasound scans. They outline your medical history and the known medical

when to expect appointments

If you are expecting your first baby and it is a single pregnancy, your appointment record should read something like this (although don't worry too much if it is a week or two different):

- ⊙ 10–12 weeks
- ⊙ 16 weeks
- ⊙ 22 weeks
- ⊙ 25 week
- ⊙ 28 weeks
- ⊙ 31 weeks
- ⊙ 34 weeks
- ⊙ 36 weeks
- ⊙ 38 weeks
- ⊙ 40 weeks
- ⊙ 41 weeks

common antenatal abbreviations

LMP last menstrual period

EDD expected date of delivery

NULLIP OR PRIMIP first baby

MULTIP more than one baby

G gravida – the number of times you have been pregnant

PARITY the number of babies delivered after 24 weeks

BP blood pressure

NAD if nothing abnormal is found in the urine

BMI body mass index

MSU mid stream specimen of urine

Rh RHESUS FACTOR Blood either has rhesus factor present (Rh+) or not (Rh-ve)

U/S ultrasound

SVD spontaneous vaginal delivery or

SVB spontaneous vaginal birth

VBAC vaginal birth after Caesarian section

Fe iron

Hb haemoglobin, or the level of iron in your blood

FH or FHHR foetal heart/foetal heart rate

FM foetal movements

PP presenting part

Vx vertex –meaning cephalic

CVS chorionic villus sample

AFP alfa-fetoprotein test

GTT glucose tolerance test

LFTs liver function test

PIH pregnancy induced hypertension

PET pre-eclampsia

APH antepartum haemorrhage or vaginal bleeding in pregnancy

Oed oedema

Palp palpation – feeling the baby in the uterus

VE vaginal examination

SPD symphysis pubis discomfort – pain in pubic bone

ECV external cephalic version (turning baby with hands from breech to head)

Cx cervix (neck of womb)

Eng engagement, or how much of your baby's head has entered the pelvis

CEPHALIC FREE the head has not entered pelvis at all

BOTTOM breech

CEPHALIC OR CEP head down

TRANSVERSE diagonally across uterus

LOA left occipito anterior

LOT left occipito transverse

LOP left occipito posterior

ROA right occipito anterior

ROL right occipito lateral

ROP right occipito posterior

DOP direct occipito posterior

DOA direct occipito anterior

RSA right sacral anterior

RSP right sacral posterior

LSA left sacral anterior

LSP left sacral posterior

history of your closest relatives. The information includes personal details, your next of kin, ethnic origin and religious beliefs. Because of the extremely personal nature of this information, you need to protect your notes.

As your pregnancy progresses, your GP, obstetrician or midwife will fill in details of your blood pressure readings, urine, the measurement of your abdomen and any issues or concerns you may raise. These are recorded alongside the date and the number of weeks pregnant you are. For example, you might see an entry that reads similar to the following:

23–5–09 (the date) 23/40 (the number of weeks pregnant you are), height of fundus (i.e. how big your abdomen is) 23cm.

Medical terms abound in obstetric notes. The table on page 119 sets out abbreviations you might find in your notes alongside their full forms, which may help you understand your notes that bit better.

THE BIRTH PLAN SECTION

The birth plan, as its name suggests, is your opportunity to write your wishes and plans for your birth. Before filling this in I suggest you read part two of this book, especially the chapter on birth plans, which is dedicated to helping you decide what you would like to put in yours. When you do come to write it, try to be comprehensive, so that whoever is looking after you gets a good idea of what you would like to happen during labour and birth.

further screening and diagnostic tests

If you needed to have tests as a result of the 12–week scan, there are some that are to be done in the first trimester (see pages 57–9). Others can only be done in the second trimester.

THE DOUBLE, TRIPLE AND QUADRUPLE TESTS (COMBINED TEST)

The tests that make up the combined test are carried out between 12 and 14 weeks. They measure hormone levels in your blood to give an estimated risk of Down's syndrome. The tests are free of charge. The double measures two markers, the triple measures three and so on.

As these screening tests are only a guide rather than definitive, you might have, say, a one in 3,000 chance of having a baby with Down's syndrome based on your results and still be that one. You can also have a one in two chance and go on to have a perfectly healthy baby. If you have a result that indicates a high chance of Down's syndrome it is important to talk through the implications with your partner and medical practitioner.

AMNIOCENTESIS

The only way of knowing for sure whether or not your baby has a chromosomal abnormality is by having an invasive diagnostic test, such as CVS (see pages 58–9) or amniocentesis. These tests carry around a 1 in 100 risk of miscarriage.

An amniocentesis can take place between 14 and 16 weeks. This test is carried out with an ultrasound scan for guidance. Your doctor will remove a

expecting more than one baby

If you are expecting twins you will already know that you are in a 'high risk' category and will have an obstetrician assigned to you. You may already know whether or not you are expecting monochorionic twins (that come from the same egg and share a placenta, also known as 'identical twins') or dichorionic twins (non-identical, usually with a placenta each).

If you are having monochorionic (identical) twins you will be monitored more closely than a mother expecting one baby and you will need to have regular scans – usually at 22 weeks, 28 weeks, 32 weeks and 36 weeks. Your doctor will probably aim to deliver your babies at around 36 weeks. Women expecting dichorionic (non-identical) twins are allowed to go to 38 weeks although, because of the increased

amount of fluid in the womb, most twins are born early.

Women expecting multiples are at higher risk of pre-eclampsia, and so need regular blood pressure and urine checks. You will also have extra blood tests to rule out anaemia, and the babies' growth will be assessed regularly to ensure it is following the expected trajectory.

Although some women don't like frequent scans, it is necessary with twins because feeling the baby's positions by hand is so much harder when there are two little bodies. The scans can also monitor the placenta function.

For more information, see also pages 59–61, and page 327 for details of services providing information on twins pregnancies.

sample of amniotic fluid from the sac around the baby using a long needle. The fluid is then tested. Your doctor will be able to tell for sure whether the baby has Down's syndrome, spina bifida or another chromosomal abnormality.

It is a good idea to take someone with you to the test for emotional as well as physical support. After the test you will be advised to rest and you may be told not to drive. If you experience severe cramping, loss of amniotic fluid or any bleeding, you need to contact your doctor immediately.

WHAT ARE THE RISKS? Both amniocentesis and CVS are invasive diagnostic tests and carry risks for your baby – you have around a 1 in 100 chance of miscarriage. Because of this, it is important to weigh up whether you are prepared to run a 1:100 risk of miscarriage for a 1:250 chance of the baby having Down's syndrome. How would you feel if you miscarried and the baby did not have a chromosomal abnormality? It's tough choice. I know women who have had a 1:25 chance of Down's syndrome who have not gone ahead with the test, and women who have had a 1:400 chance who have had the test. Every woman is different.

When you receive a result of 1:250 or less, you are immediately offered amniocentesis or CVS. My advice is think very carefully about the consequences before you take the decision. Some women find they are at odds with their partner over their decision, which can present a double dilemma. (See page 327 for sources of information about and support during antenatal testing.)

the 20-week scan (anomoly scan)

Your next scan will be between 20 and 22 weeks. The sonographer (the person qualified to carry out an ultrasound scan) will be looking at your baby from top-to-toe externally to check everything is normal. They will also check your baby's internal body, looking particularly at the heart, bladder, brain, spine and position of the lungs, as well as the blood flow from the placenta to the baby.

Some couples are so preoccupied with finding out the sex or getting a print out of the new baby that they forget that this is an important scan for checking the wellbeing and growth of your baby. It's worth being quietly aware that there are abnormalities that can show up on these scans (see below), but that the vast majority of babies will be growing normally. Approximately 10% of scans need to be repeated for one reason or another.

SHOULD WE FIND OUT THE SEX?

Approximately 60% of couples now find out the sex of their baby. It's worth giving this some thought in advance. Chat through your views with your partner – you may have different ideas on this. Some couples decide that one will find out and the other won't.

And remember, as always, to expect the unexpected. It may be that you both want to know the sex, but that the baby has different ideas and won't give up the secret because of the position he or she is lying in.

WHAT MIGHT THE SCAN REVEAL?

Occasionally couples can discover their baby has an abnormality at the 20-week scan. This can be at best slightly worrying and, in rare cases, devastating. Some couples like to discuss this possibility in advance; others believe dwelling on the negatives can be unnecessarily upsetting for women at what is usually such a happy and blossoming time of pregnancy.

ABNORMALITIES Common abnormalities that are detected on the 20-week scan include:

⊙ cleft palate with or without cleft lip, which can be indicative of something more profound
⊙ six toes – this, again, can be indicative of a genetic problem, but is also hereditary
⊙ talipes, or 'club foot' – this can be a symptom of something more complicated, but your baby can otherwise be perfectly healthy. 'Club foot' can be corrected with surgery after birth
⊙ heart abnormalities – there are a whole range of heart abnormalities that can be picked up on a 20-week scan which will require you to be referred to a specialist hospital. Yours will no longer be categorized as a normal pregnancy. Your consultant will talk you through your options
⊙ exomphalus, which is a defect in the abdominal wall whereby the inner organs are exposed to the outside of the skin. This often means that the baby will need to be delivered by C-section, but regardless of the way he or she is born, they will need to be immediately transferred to a neo-natal

unit, and surgery will follow shortly afterwards

⊙ missing limbs or shortening of a limb – again this can be a problem on its own, or a symptom of another problem.

In cases where an abnormality is picked up, parents are offered counselling with a specialist. You will probably be shown photographs of cases so that you know what to expect when your child is born and what to expect after surgery. You will be given the opportunity to meet other mothers who have gone through a similar situation, as well as specialist nurses, surgeons and so on. All this will happen in advance of your baby's birth.

gestational diabetes

In the pregnant population, 2% of women will develop gestational diabetes when they have not previously been diabetic. Diabetes is a condition where blood sugar levels remain high due to reduced insulin (a hormone that breaks down sugar). Gestational diabetes occurs when the pancreas is unable to produce enough insulin due to hormonal changes and the demands of the unborn baby. The condition normally develops around 28 weeks and goes away after birth. Women most at risk are those who:

⊙ have a family history of diabetes or whose mothers had gestational diabetes
⊙ have previously had a baby over 4.5kg (10lb)
⊙ are overweight
⊙ have previously had a stillborn baby
⊙ are overweight
⊙ are carrying twins.

Symptoms of gestational diabetes are increased thirst, tiredness and needing to pee more often.

If you are at risk you will be offered a routine test called a glucose-tolerance test at 28–30 weeks. If your blood sugar levels are raised, you will be referred for dietary advice and to be taught how to test yourself. In rare instances, insulin injections are required. Ultrasound checks will be done to check the baby's weight and amniotic fluid levels. NICE (the National Institute for Clinical Excellence) do not recommend routine screening for all pregnant women, but some midwives test for sugar in urine at routine antenatal visits and will take matters further if sugar is seen in the urine. After birth, your baby's blood sugar level will be checked regularly. You will need to ensure that your baby feeds regularly to prevent hypoglycaemia (low blood sugar).

You may also be offered further genetic tests to see if the abnormality detected on the scan is a lone problem or if there are further abnormalities. Your obstetrician will try to get the whole picture. That said, the majority of abnormalities are a one-off and unexplained. In rare cases there can be grave problems that will affect the baby's chances of survival and you may be confronted with difficult decisions. (See Expecting the Unexpected, pages 264–79.)

In some cases the 20-week scan may reveal very common issues that need to be monitored.

A 'LOW-LYING' PLACENTA OR PLACENTA PRAEVIA This means that your placenta is close to or partially covers your cervix (the baby's exit route). In the vast majority of these cases, the placenta will move as the uterus expands, rather like the dot on a balloon that is being inflated.

You will need another scan between 32 and 34 weeks if you have a 'low-lying placenta'. By 32 weeks only 1% of those diagnosed at 20 weeks are still praevia. If at 34 weeks your placenta still covers or partially covers your cervix, or if the placenta remains too low to risk a natural birth, you will be given a scheduled Caesarean section a week or two weeks before your due date. In the event that you experience any painless bleeding – a symptom of placenta praevia – you may be admitted to hospital for monitoring. Your doctor may also recommend that you take bed rest.

INCREASED AMNIOTIC FLUID This can be very common and is not always a cause for concern. However, your doctor will want to make sure that the baby is swallowing properly. He or she will also want to exclude any signs of gestational diabetes, especially with bigger babies.

'SMALL FOR GESTATIONAL AGE' This used to be known as 'small for dates'. During your antenatal check-ups your doctor or midwife will feel your abdomen and measure its size in centimetres to check the baby's growth. If growth starts to tail off – and there is usually concern if the baby is three centimetres less than the corresponding number of weeks – then you will be sent for an ultrasound. I should say here that it is not always a matter for concern.

This scan will be able to check:

⊙ the volume of amniotic fluid around the baby
⊙ the measurement of the baby's head
⊙ the measurement of the baby's tummy.

From the results, your doctor will be able to work out the estimated foetal weight (EFW). Scans are the most accurate way to diagnose a baby that is small for gestational age (SGA). You may then be scheduled for regular scans to check the baby is growing along its own trajectory, even if that is smaller than usual. In many cases, the obstetrician will be satisfied that the baby is growing perfectly well. It may be, however, that he or she has concerns. They will want to check that the placenta and umbilical cord are functioning properly and that the baby is getting the nutrients he or she needs. In this case you will be scheduled for an earlier delivery date.

A baby that is small for gestational age runs an increased risk of stillbirth, lack of oxygen at birth (hypoxia), neonatal complications and impaired brain development. (See page 327 for sources of further information.)

Expectant women who smoke should be given information about the effects on their pregnancy and given help and support to stop.

antenatal classes

It's wise to book now for antenatal classes as they do tend to book up well in advance. Most women start antenatal classes at around 30 weeks and attend at least four classes. There are various options available, from evening to weekend classes. Some are free and others need to be booked privately.

These classes are a fantastic place to air questions and fears, as well as to learn crucial information.

NCT

The most well-established body for birthing classes is the National Childbirth Trust (NCT), which has been operational since the 1950s. It's an excellent body and charity, and in addition to running nationwide classes that are a great source for information, the NCT also organize breastfeeding groups and get-togethers for new mums and their babies. See page 328 for contact details for the NCT.

Do book your birth classes well in advance, especially in London, as they book up quickly. You will be amazed at how much you value these classes, not just because of the information they provide but the friends you can make.

HOSPITAL-BASED CLASSES

Many maternity hospitals offer courses run by hospital midwives. For example I run one at Queen Charlotte's. These groups are often small and partners are very much encouraged to attend.

GP

Your GP clinic may also offer classes, but if not they will be able to put you in touch with a local group.

RETREATS

Some organizations run 'birth preparation weekends' that both expectant parents can attend, and where you will meet other parents-to-be.

preparing your mind for birth

If there is one thing I hear myself saying more than anything else at work, it's: 'You can do it!' So often in our lives we are confronted with things we would like to try, but shy away from them because we think we can't do it. An immediate example that springs to mind is a marathon. We think, 'That's something other people do. I can't possibly do that!' But have we just opted out of something we could have done with a bit of physical and mental preparation? This is so true of the marathon of labour.

empowerment

Although many women today still start pregnancy afraid of birth, an increasing number are recognizing they have a part to play in the process. You have a choice about what course your birth will take. You can take control and manage your own journey. Empowerment is all about 'making your head stronger than

developing your own visualisation

If you have followed the guidance for establishing a personal visualisation on page 72, you should now have a detailed picture of a mental sanctuary. During this trimester, bring your senses into the scene.

Return to your special place and look around you. What can you smell? The fresh grass, clean air, flowers? Now what can you feel? The sun on your face, the crisp fresh air against your cheeks, the grass beneath your feet, the soft silky sand between your toes, a sun umbrella gently flapping, chattering in the distance, the wonderful feeling of cool sea and warm sun? And what can you hear? The rustling of leaves, the wind whistling through a window, birds singing, a cockerel crowing loudly, water trickling and slowly dripping? Consider how everything continues in its own time and space, and enjoy the wonderful moments of just being alive and healthy.

Practise bringing your senses into your scene in this way, so that it becomes more and more 'real'.

your uterus' – that is, making mental preparation an essential part of looking towards your birth (see pages 71–3). This option is available for almost everyone – yes, even those who are very high risk and are chalked in for a Caesarean early on. You can still enjoy your pregnancy; you can still have natural elements in your birth. It's all about the way you view it.

Try out all the options for pregnancy – yoga, walks in the park, planning with your partner. Try out the visualisations (see opposite and pages 72 and 168), even if your first reaction was 'Isn't this a load of dippy rubbish?'. I've seen the results and I wouldn't write about it if it wasn't worth it!

Enjoy the feeling of looking forward to the next chapter in your life, the chapter with you and your little baby. Enjoy planning ahead. Many of the techniques I am teaching you now are invaluable for life with children.

For birth, try to concentrate on the 'I can' approach. Really think through your options. Take in the information. Think of the comforting things that underpin the birth (see pages 236–240). The message I want to get across to each and every mother is that the marathon of labour is something you too can be involved in. You can have a positive birth. You can feel empowered.

THINGS TO THINK ABOUT

⊙ The second trimester is a wonderful opportunity for you to feel positive about your pregnancy, your birth and your life ahead with the new baby. Relish this time.

⊙ It's a great time to make plans for your birth. While the event is still a long way off, you have plenty of time to think about it and consider what feels right and what doesn't. Start a programme of mental and physical preparation now – it's a great investment.

⊙ Have you thought about what will happen after the birth? Sort through what you want in terms of help in the early weeks. What will the baby need? It's time to start shopping for the baby.

⊙ It's also a great time for practical preparation in life in general. Do you have financial concerns? Work concerns? Concerns with family and friends? These are all issues that you can deal with now.

⊙ You can use this time to read, relax and enjoy thinking about this incredible time of your life.

third trimester weeks 26–40

You are nearing the end of pregnancy and you may be starting to slow down physically as you get heavier (although that doesn't stop many women making manic last minute preparations). You are probably thinking more and more about the birth and preparing for the arrival of the baby. You may feel a lot more interested in the finer details of birth and find yourself gripped by television or websites that deal with birth. You may also find yourself thinking more and more about the reality of life with a newborn baby.

coping with physical changes

Some of the pregnancy complaints in the third trimester are very similar to the first or second trimester and, where that occurs, I provide page references so you can flip back to the relevant sections.

STRETCH MARKS

You may have felt jubilant about not having had stretch marks up until this point, only to find that they suddenly appear a few days before giving birth. If that is the case, try to remember that it's a small price to pay for a beautiful baby. We all experience one symptom or another – no one gets away scot-free. (See also page 86.)

LEG AND FOOT CRAMPS

Cramps can be caused by a number of factors, including excessively stretched ligaments and muscles and decreased circulation to the legs (exacerbated by sitting for long periods and flying). Your heart, kidneys and your circulatory system are worked extremely hard to help you function as normal during the last weeks of pregnancy, but the weight of the uterus puts pressure on the nerves connecting the trunk to the legs, which causes muscles in your legs to seize up.

If you are suffering from sudden cramps, especially in the middle of the night, you'll know that they can be so severe that you are left with an aching sensation the following morning. Some women find it impossible to stay still and hobble out of bed in agony. If you can't sit down, get to a wall, lean forward into it with one knee bent and the other straight and try a lunging position. I recommend that women who suffer from leg cramps do this every night before they go to bed anyway. Try to alternate exercise with rest – and elevate your legs and feet when you can.

If the cramp is in your foot, put pressure on the area with your thumbs. Try to massage the pain. If it's unbearable, perhaps ask your partner to massage the area while you try to stretch it as much as possible.

A hot compress – or hot water bottle – may help relieve the pain by relaxing the muscle that is in spasm. To prevent further attacks, you can alternate a heat treatment (hot bath or hot water bottle) before bed, with a cold compress (ice wrapped in a tea towel) used for up to 10 minutes, three or four times a day.

Tight socks, shoes and clothing can make cramp worse. You should also avoid standing for too long and sitting with your legs crossed. (See also the advice on pages 91–2.)

Cramp can be a sign that you are deficient in potassium and calcium, which is why the remedy of 'a banana before bed' is so widely quoted. Increase your intake of the following foods if you suffer from cramp. It may help.

Calcium-rich foods include:
- dairy products (yoghurt, milk and cheese especially)
- tofu
- fish (salmon and sardines are good choices as they are also good sources of potassium)
- vegetables (try greens, broccoli, peas, sprouts, pak choi and okra)
- nuts and seeds (almonds and sesame seeds are also good sources of potassium)
- Pulses (go for white beans and baked beans).

Potassium-rich foods include:
- cereals (choose bran-based cereals, such as All Bran or Bran Flakes)
- nuts and seeds (most nuts and seeds are potassium-rich)
- fruit (bananas, figs, dried apricots, sultanas, raisins, dates, grapefruits and oranges are good choices, although bear in mind that citrus fruits can exacerbate acid indigestion)
- fish (go for pilchards and sardines)
- vegetables (try baked potatoes with the skin on)
- dairy products (yoghurt and cottage cheese are potassium-rich)
- carbohydrates (try wholemeal pasta and wheat germ).

RESTLESS LEG SYNDROME (RLS)

Less common than leg cramps, RLS is a neurological condition that can also affect pregnant women. The basic symptom is the uncontrollable urge to move your leg, but you may also experience itching or a 'creepy crawly' sensation. Your leg may even jolt or spasm. Once you have moved, however, the urge reoccurs, leading to a frustrating and sleepless night.

In pregnancy, RLS is caused by the restrictions on your blood circulation, although it will be exacerbated by stress, tension, caffeine, chocolate, alcohol and smoking. Alternating hot and cold packs on the areas is one way to treat RLS. Another is massage. Perhaps ask your partner to massage your legs before you sleep to improve circulation. A hot bath (although not too hot in pregnancy), with your legs propped up above your heart, may also help improve the condition. It should also help you relax. Try a couple of drops of lavender oil in the water, too.

If you are suffering badly from RLS you need to see your GP who may prescribe medication, or recommend that you take certain vitamins or minerals that are safe in pregnancy and suitable for your individual needs. (See page 328 for details of a service providing information on RLS.)

STRETCHING PAIN

A general softening and relaxing of the muscles and ligaments in pregnancy allows your body to stretch. This is both to make room for your bump, and also in preparation for birth. As the weight of your baby increases, however, the relaxed muscles and ligaments feel the strain, and you may experience stretching pain in the groin area or around the bump. Much like leg cramps,

elasticated belts or pregnancy girdles

I cannot recommend these enough. Many women have described pregnancy girdles as a godsend. They come in many forms but the best ones are the very wide elasticated belts that wrap around you and are fastened with thick Velcro strips. They provide support for the bump in the shape of a sling, but should really be fitted by a specialist.

Wearing a pregnancy girdle can stop all those stretching, tweaking pains that you may start to feel around the sides of your tummy as the bump gets bigger.

They can provide great support for weak or strained backs and also stop you from twisting and bending in awkward positions.

A cheaper alternative is the do-it-yourself wide scarf (a thin one may be better in summer) which you can wrap around you and tie under your bump like a belt. Both these versions of the belt can be really helpful if you like to walk but the stretching pains are making it difficult. (See page 329 for sources of pregnancy girdles.)

the stretching pain some women experience can be agony. It is almost as if you can feel each ligament tugging as you move.

You need to be conscious of good posture in order to give your overworked body some balance. Try not to bend too far forward or back and avoid the trademark pregnancy waddle. Also be conscious of your centre of gravity.

The first remedy is to sleep surrounded by pillows to prevent awkward turns in your sleep. Try to keep your back relatively straight, but lodge a pillow in every crevice until you are literally buoyed up by them. Some women additionally use the V-shaped pillows that are also good for breastfeeding later, but others just find them annoying.

If you feel your ligaments pulling during the day, when you are walking or trying to reach for something, you might find a pregnancy girdle (see box, page 133) useful. These are wide elasticated belts that provide support for the bump and can serve to remind you not to twist too much.

If you start to feel the pressure of baby weight pushing down into your pubic area – a sensation that has been described by one mother as 'my bits being pushed down to my knees', then you are doing too much and need to rest. Walking may help to relieve the symptoms, but it is not good for you if you feel too much pain, or that 'down to your knees' feeling.

SCIATICA

Sciatica is the sharp pain, tingling or even numbness that you may feel around your bottom, hips and thighs. It's caused by the weight of your uterus on the sciatic nerve. In most cases sciatica is just another annoying side-effect of pregnancy, but if the pain travels lower than your buttocks into your leg it can be more serious and so should be reported to your midwife or doctor.

The most effective relief for sciatica is heat in the form of a hot bath or hot compress. Also, try to not to sleep on the area that is causing the pain. (See also the advice on page 92.)

SYMPHYSIS PUBIS DYSFUNCTION (SPD)

Around 10% of women suffer from symphysis pubis dysfunction and it can be excruciating. Women often report it towards the end of the second trimester and the beginning of the third trimester and in the last few weeks. I'm sorry to say that if you had it in a first pregnancy you are likely to get it in subsequent pregnancies. You may first notice it as searing pain in the groin, especially when you move your legs apart. In pronounced cases women say they experience a 'grinding or clicking' feeling in the pubic area.

SPD occurs when the two sections of your pelvis meet a fibrous band that is interlaced with ligaments. Normally this area, the symphysis pubis joint, is not exposed to movement. During pregnancy, however, it is susceptible to the same hormonal changes that allow your other muscles and ligaments to relax in preparation for childbirth.

Below is the advice I give to women with SPD:

- think 'knees together, knees together' when you are doing anything that involves separating your legs – like getting out of the car or swinging out of bed
- where you have to separate your legs, such as when you're walking, getting dressed, climbing the stairs or getting in and out of the bath, do so very carefully, using your stronger leg first
- a pregnancy girdle (see page 133) may provide some relief
- swimming can be hugely helpful, although be careful of breaststroke – the frog's leg action will really exacerbate the pain
- don't lift anything too heavy – shopping bags can cause pain – and be careful of strenuous pushing. I have had women who found that pushing an older child in the buggy or supermarket trolleys caused them pain
- rest more, but make sure you are well supported by pillows or cushions
- use a Tubigrip – this is a stretchy elasticated seamless bandage which you can buy from specialist chemists for different parts of the body. The abdominal size can be pulled up over your legs and then over your tummy and you can wear clothes over the top.
- make sure you go to the loo often – if you have a full bladder it can cause increased pressure over the symphysis pubic bone causing even more discomfort
- wear comfortable, loose, stretchy clothing – no tight jeans or tight belts
- don't forget to do your pelvic floor exercises (see pages 37–8), and try to do a little exercise often.

You need to let your midwife or doctor know if you suspect you have SPD. He or she can refer you to a physiotherapist if necessary. SPD may also have implications for your birth. I usually suggest that the left lateral position (lying on your left side with your knees bent towards your chest as much as possible, with the upper leg supported by a birth attendant) is best for birth.

BACKACHE

Backache is one of those symptoms of pregnancy that seems to straddle all trimesters and affects nearly all women at one time or other – about 10% suffer very badly. I have already touched on the subject on pages 82–4, where you'll find more advice on dealing with backache.

By the third trimester, it's not just hormones, softening ligaments and your muscles becoming more elastic that is causing your back to ache, but the sheer weight of the bump on your front. If you are suffering badly you may even have adopted that pigeon-like shuffle when you walk, which you need to try and correct by standing up straight with your shoulders down. Don't lock your knees when you're standing.

Many women feel the pain concentrated in the sacroiliac joint at the base of the spine – a weight-bearing joint that has been working hard during pregnancy, particularly if you have other small children who demand to be carried, transferred in and out of cots and baths etc.

There is also some anecdotal evidence that a bad previous birth or a badly administered epidural can result in lower back pain during subsequent pregnancies. The pain can feel worse during Braxton Hicks contractions when your uterus tightens and the pain drops low, even into your back passage.

While these tips for relieving backache (see left) may help in the short term, you probably need to introduce other measures to help support your expanding bump. For example: practise good posture; exercise –

tips for relieving back pain

One fabulous thing about back pain remedies is that they can bring immediate relief. Try the following:

- ⊙ do the cat stretch (see page 82)
- ⊙ lie on your back and bring your legs up to your chest (around your bump!). Hug your legs and rock gently on your spine and sacrum as if you were massaging it with the floor. Do this exercise on a mat, a rug or on carpeted floor (as opposed to the bed, which doesn't give you the right support)
- ⊙ use a pregnancy girdle (see page 133), which may bring you some relief
- ⊙ hold a hot compress, in the form of a hot water bottle, against the affected area for fast relief
- ⊙ ask your doctor to refer you to an osteopath.

swimming and yoga are good choices; take care when you lift other children (see pages 83–4 for tips on protecting your back when picking up toddlers); try not to stay in the same position for too long – especially sitting down; avoid soft chairs and sofas – it is better to sit on the floor; avoid bucket seats; and sleep on your left side, propped up with pillows.

The good news is that the vast majority of back complaints clear up shortly after the baby arrives.

SHORTNESS OF BREATH

Almost all women experience shortness of breath in the last trimester, regardless of how fit they are, because the expanding uterus is putting pressure on the diaphragm. Merely climbing a short flight of stairs may leave you suddenly short of breath and panting for air. Don't worry, however – the lack of oxygen you feel doesn't affect the baby, and this pregnancy symptom will disappear once you give birth.

It may sound like a paradox, but your breathing can actually be improved by gentle exercise. Good posture helps, as does propping yourself with pillows while you sleep, which allows the pressure to be taken off your diaphragm.

INCREASED NEED TO PEE

These twice or three times nightly trips to the loo are caused by the increased weight of the uterus on your bladder. As the baby descends and the head moves lower down the pelvis, you may feel the need to go even more frequently.

You need to be organized when planning long journeys, meetings or going to events where a loo isn't close at hand. It's really not recommended to hold urine in for too long because you are at an increased risk of urinary infection while you're pregnant. If there is an occasion where you know you're not going to be able to get to the loo quickly, your only course of action may be to limit your fluid intake (although this is not recommended regularly and you must be careful not to get dehydrated).

HEARTBURN

This can be a real problem in the last trimester and, combined with the fact that your uterus is pushing against your stomach, it can lead to an overall slowing down of your appetite if you think you are going to have an attack.

On pages 81–2 I give tips to relieve heartburn, but one tip I will add here is that you should try to eat as slowly as possible. Chew every mouthful thoroughly before swallowing. Rushing your food can set off a crippling episode and I know women who have suffered so badly in the third trimester that they have ended up sleeping with a bottle of Gaviscon next to the bed.

MORNING SICKNESS

Some women say that they start feeling sick again in the final trimester and, in rare cases, it's possible to have third trimester morning sickness. In the first trimester, nausea is caused by a huge increase in hormones. In the third trimester, pregnancy-related sickness (as opposed to a bug or food poisoning) is far more likely to be caused by indigestion (see above) or tiredness (see below), although certain foods can trigger sickness, such as fruit.

You can experience nausea and vomiting as part of the onset of labour (see pages 233–4.)

TIREDNESS

Tiredness now doesn't feel quite as debilitating as the knockout fatigue of trimester one, but you will still appreciate an early night and, if you can, a lunchtime nap. First-trimester tiredness is predominantly caused by hormones – progesterone is thought to have a sedative effect. Now the reasons for tiredness are more obvious: you are carrying a large weight around all day and providing the growing baby with more nutrition than at any time to date.

As always, listen to your body. If you feel exhausted by 9pm, go to bed. Avoid the urge to pack too much into your day – be it for work, house renovations or organizing last minute preparations for the baby.

Those who have other children or a busy job and can't afford the luxury of a midday nap need to be resourceful. Does your company have an office-based nurse? Can you ask to use her room for a nap? Can you get grandma or a neighbour in to help out with the kids while you conk out for an hour? Perhaps you could even encourage an older child to have a nap with you. How about weekends? Can you catch up on your sleep then? Try to schedule a rest period into your day.

BRAXTON HICKS

John Braxton Hicks was a Victorian doctor who first described these 'painless' uterine contractions, which are often called 'practice contractions'. I have touched on Braxton Hicks in The Second Trimester (see page 91), but you will probably notice them more in the third trimester. They are characterized by a sudden tightening of the uterus, which may appear square and hard to the touch. They are nothing to be concerned about and happen intermittently from the beginning of the second trimester, although they are increasingly noticeable as your bump gets bigger.

The tightening of the uterus, particularly in second or subsequent pregnancies, may also be a little uncomfortable, tug a little or even cause discomfort in the back passage, although Braxton Hicks shouldn't be painful as such. Any discomfort should subside when you move around. If you are experiencing continuing pain, or if you are having regular runs of four 'contractions' every hour, however, you need to contact your midwife to rule out preterm labour.

After 37 weeks, you may notice that the runs of Braxton Hicks become more regular. For some women, bursts of 'practice contractions' become more intense. This is sometimes called 'pre-labour'. Others are unsure if they are in labour or not. One way to tell is by changing position, moving around or by having a warm bath. If it is 'false labour' the contractions should go away. For others, the Braxton Hicks are entirely unnoticeable and they have no indication of a labour contraction until labour starts.

OEDEMA

Most women have a little swelling in the second or third trimesters. See page 84 to find tips for reducing swelling. If pressing on the skin leaves an indentation it might be a cause for concern, so speak to your doctor or midwife.

NIGHT WAKING

From as early as 32 weeks, you may find you are waking up in the middle of the night. In some cases this is because of the need to pee, in others it is because of how difficult it has become to turn over at night with a large bump. Sometimes, however, it seems inexplicable.

Some obstetricians and childbirth specialists have put this down to the body preparing for interrupted nights of sleep when you are breastfeeding and this sounds like a logical suggestion to me. Pregnant women find themselves doing and feeling some seemingly strange things in the last trimester, from crazy nesting to feelings of sudden loneliness (see below).

SUDDEN FEELING OF LONELINESS

Women often report this under-researched area of late pregnancy. Some find it difficult and unpleasant, others enjoy and even indulge it by switching off their phone and spending more time alone at home or on long walks.

My colleague Yehudi Gordon believes these sudden moments of loneliness are nature's way of preparing you for the highs and lows of motherhood[10]. The early days of motherhood, while utterly joyful, can also bring long periods of loneliness, particularly at night. While your baby is small and relatively uncommunicative, and the fuss of the new arrival has died down, you may find yourself spending more time on your own than you ever have before.

It may be worth thinking about how you will spend your time as a new mother, particularly if you have moved to a new area. Now is a good time to look into mother and baby groups. Contact the Meet a Mum Association to find other mothers who may feel the same (see page 328 for contact details).

EXTREME MOOD SWINGS

Doctors may tell you that mood swings in the first trimester of pregnancy are worse than later on, but in my experience I have found the reverse – that in the late weeks of pregnancy, during which the mother feels tired and heavy, mood swings can be far greater than the blips of early pregnancy.

As the pregnancy comes to a close women report feeling very subdued one moment and angry the next. The waiting game of 'when will the baby arrive?' is aggravated by everyone asking if the baby has arrived. While the mood swings are part of a natural process, they can also be the modern woman's way of dealing with what is at once the most fantastic event of her life, and also something of a crisis. Many women feel 'I'm fed up and I want this baby to come now', and at the exact same moment, 'How am I going to cope? I've got months of no sleep ahead of me and I'm already at my wits end.'

The sense of anticipation while you wait for the major life events of labour, childbirth, meeting, getting to know and caring for your baby, can be suffocating. Women often find themselves taking on immense challenges shortly before birth in an effort to feel in control. It's not uncommon, for example, to clear out the attic, reorganize the kitchen or decide that the garden needs an overhaul.

As I've said so often throughout the book, the key to coping is patience. You have to sit back and take a clichéd deep breath and try to relax. (See my tips on relaxation techniques on pages 73–4.) If you want to clear out the attic, go ahead. You could consiously see it as an act of clearing out your old life to make way for the new. Just don't exhaust yourself. Working on the garden might be just the distraction you need. You could see the planting of new bulbs as part of the life cycle you are involved in, too. You may find these thoughts give you ideas for your visualisations during labour.

All these activities are commendable if they are done as part of an exercise in being calm and relaxed, rather than in a state of frenzy.

NESTING

The nesting instinct (in the form of spring cleaning, planning, the urge to repaint the house, etc.) is an urge that is entirely natural when you are coming to the end of your pregnancy. Some people see it as a sign that labour is approaching. There is very little you can do to stop it so my words of advice are:

⊙ try not to overdo it and make yourself so exhausted you can't cope with labour
⊙ be cautious when handling chemical cleaners and paint fumes.

Like mood swings, you may find the urge to clean and nest seizes you unexpectedly, for example when you were about to sit down and have a relaxing evening in front of the TV. You may also find that pregnancy indecision combined with the urge to nest produces some extreme results. One mother I know insisted on decorating the whole house shortly before the birth of her son. She chose a colour for the sitting room, but once on the walls she decided she hated it. Her husband tried to reassure her but she was adamant that it had to be changed. When this didn't look like it would happen immediately, she became very agitated. In the middle of the night her husband woke up to find his wife had left the bed. He wearily went to look for her. He found her, roller in hand and with a triumphant grin, in the sitting room. The walls had been returned to white.

preparing your body for birth

If you haven't yet exercised during your pregnancy, it's not too late to start. You will feel the benefits in this trimester, as your body becomes larger and you feel less comfortable. If you spend much of your day at a desk, it's even more important to try and fit in a swim or a walk, even if it's the last thing you feel like when you get home from work. Not only will it help you feel better, but toning up your muscles will help you during labour. There are other things you can do, too, to prepare for labour, such as perineal massage and using alternative therapies to relax your body or turn a breech baby.

exercise

WALKING

Walking is great for getting rid of that 'creaky' feeling that comes from sitting at a desk for long periods. It can help lift low moods and improve circulation, help with breathlessness and is generally beneficial to your health. It's also a lovely way to enjoy your time with your partner or friends and gives you a good opportunity to chat about the coming changes in your life.

In all four of my pregnancies, I used London's parks and walked around, taking in the scenery, watching the families and contemplating how my baby would fit into my life. Walking can be a great release. It helps to put things in perspective and blows away any cobwebs that have settled from spending too long in the house or in the office.

I know so many women who have spent almost the entirety of the maternity leave out on walks and it has really helped them during labour. One lady talked about going to watch the little boats on the pond in a park near her house. She went every day and watched as the boats, with their numbered sails, bobbed from one side of the pond to the other. Quite unconsciously, this image came to her during labour and became her visualisation. During each contraction she would imagine she was blowing the sail of a boat to help it to the other side. She counted her breaths by imagining the number on the sail, and averaged then breaths per contraction: ten little boats blown to the other side of the pond. Another lady enjoyed riverside walks and imagined being beside the water and listening to the gentle trickle while rocking her new baby in her arms.

Some women, however, find walking near impossible in the later stages of pregnancy, especially if the baby's head gets too low and you are experiencing the tweaks and twinges of the last few weeks. If that is the case, and using a pregnancy girdle (see page 133) isn't helping, I recommend you try something else rather than give up on exercise altogether.

SWIMMING

It's never too late to start swimming and it can be surprisingly welcome later in pregnancy, even if you haven't dipped your big toe in a pool for some years. When I suggest swimming, many women immediately ask, 'But where can I get a swimming costume that fits?' The answer is that they are readily available. You can buy maternity swimwear from Mothercare and John Lewis, as well as a number of websites. Don't worry about how you will look – no one is judging you, and the important thing to concentrate on is how you will feel after a lovely, calming, gentle swim.

At the end of pregnancy there are times when you feel like a heifer – everything is huge, you feel ungainly and you are limited to a snail's pace. I remember feeling the weight of the entire pregnancy moving south – especially with my fourth pregnancy when I felt my stomach muscles had given up altogether and I had to almost gather my bump in my arms in order to move. That said, any exercise helps, both mentally and physically. It helps you build up your stamina, which is essential for labour, and can help you avoid putting on excess weight.

The water keeps you cool, provides natural support for the baby and will give you a feeling of freedom from the bump. While you can practise most swimming strokes in the early months of pregnancy, you may find something simpler works in the third trimester.

Some osteopaths believe breaststroke can exacerbate back problems, but you can certainly enjoy a gentle backstroke as long as you don't feel the pressure of your baby weight too heavily. You can also swim on your front holding a float while kicking your legs behind you. This is great for improving circulation in the lower part of your body.

My advice is to steer clear of the fast lane, even if you are a seasoned swimmer, because flying limbs and strong kicks can be a threat to your bump. I would also avoid tumble turns as it can exacerbate acid indigestion.

I have looked after women who swam even in early labour – one did 100 lengths and only just made it to the hospital in time for the birth. Don't swim, however, if your waters have broken, because of the risk of infection.

YOGA

Many women don't even start yoga classes until they have reached the third trimester, so don't worry about being too late to pick it up. Pregnancy yoga is a particularly gentle and calming strain of the discipline, but some women find it too 'slow and boring' if they attend classes too early in pregnancy. They say that you really reap the benefits later in pregnancy when it can be the one thing you really look forward to in a week.

Yoga is a great all-round exercise – it helps with circulation, breathing, stretching and eliminating many of the aches and pains caused by the minor disorders of pregnancy. It also teaches you how to retreat into a quiet space and shut out the outside world – a lesson that is invaluable for labour.

massaging the perineum

The perineum is the area of skin between the vulva and the anus. It is made up of skin, fat and muscle that will stretch to allow the baby's head to crown before birth. Approximately 85% of women suffer 'trauma to the perineum' during birth, and 60–70% need stitches (see pages 261–3).

Perineal massage can reduce the risk of tearing and having an episiotomy. It stretches the area prior to birth, making the tissues more elastic and less susceptible to tearing. It also allows you to become familiar with the 'stinging sensation' you will experience just before birth. Without this familiarity, it can be a moment of panic for some women who chose to labour without drugs.

Perineal massage used to be a practice very much confined to the Natural Birth Movement. If I had suggested it in a birth preparation class even 10 years ago, it would probably have been met by expressions of faint revulsion. Even midwives were sceptical in the early days. The anecdotal success of perineal massage, however, means that it has been accepted in the mainstream and is now frequently recommended. Statistically, it's thought that you can reduce your chance of tearing by up to 10% by doing your perineal massage for 10 minutes a day in the last four or five weeks of pregnancy.

This can be an opportunity to get your partner involved – especially as the expanse of bump can make the massage awkward for you to do. However, some women prefer to do the perineal massage themselves.

HOW TO DO A PERINEAL MASSAGE

To make the area soft and elastic it's best to do the massage after a warm bath, but not essential. If you haven't bathed, make sure you wash your hands and find somewhere warm and relaxed to do the massage. You will need a massage oil – I recommend olive oil, but you can use sweet almond oil or any of the 'preconditioned' or baby massage oils on the market – or a lubricant that is not petroleum-based. If you're alone, it's probably best to do the first few attempts with a mirror (it's hard to see over the bump).

Find somewhere comfortable to sit with your legs apart. Insert your thumbs into the vagina and push out the sides for a count of 10 (building up to 50) and then gently massage up and down with your thumbs in a 'U' shape. Using your thumbs, gently pull the tissue forwards – this simulates the feeling of the baby's head coming down during birth. Move your thumbs down towards your bottom and gently stretch the area until you feel a sharp, tingling sensation – it's the same burning sensation you get from pulling the sides of your mouth apart with your index fingers. Hold the stretch until it stops burning, then gently massage the area with your thumbs (or thumb and index finger), again in a 'U' shape.

Be careful not to be too vigorous with the massage or you could cause swelling or bruising. The more you practise, the easier the stretch will feel.

It's worth holding on to the idea that the feeling that you get from a perineal stretch is very similar to the feeling of the baby's head pressing down, as it may allow you to be more relaxed in the event. If you have an epidural, you won't feel the same stinging sensation because the anaesthetic will numb the area. You should, however, feel the intense pressure bearing down, and that allows you to have some control in the pushing stage.

alternative therapies

ACUPUNCTURE

Acupuncture is a Far Eastern practice that has been used for 2,500 years to treat medical complaints, pain and to promote generall wellbeing. Your therapist will use fine needles to stimulate 'acupoints' on different parts of the body. Mostly this is painless and you may not even feel the needle go in. However, on the bonier points of your legs, it might be a tiny bit sore.

Antenatal acupuncture by a trained practitioner is fabulous in the last few weeks of pregnancy when it can help your body prepare for labour. Women have reported 'feeling their cervix opening and effacing' shortly after a session. You can also use acupuncture for induction (which has differing results).

A type of acupuncture called moxibustion is often recommended for turning breech babies (heat is used by the little toe, rather than needles), and I have heard anecdotally that this has quite a good success rate. I also know of a study that showed that acupuncture before labour reduced the need for epidural analgesia and the women assessed were significantly more relaxed.

Others have promoted the use of acupuncture during labour, both to regulate contractions and reduce pain, and for fast expulsion of the placenta.

REFLEXOLOGY

Reflexology has to be one of the most enjoyable therapies in late pregnancy. You will usually lie on your back, propped up by pillows, while the therapist sets about massaging key areas of your feet. The idea is that different organs in your body correspond to zones on your feet and, in a process of massaging, squeezing and pressing, a therapist can help drain 'blockages' in these zones.

Not only does it feel wonderful to have someone manipulate your poor, tired hardworking feet, it also has serious health benefits. It has been shown to be an

raspberry leaf tea

Raspberry leaf tea is said to tone your uterus in preparation for labour and there are many women who believe it can shorten the second stage by making the contractions 'more effective'. Some therapists advise against drinking it before the 34th week of pregnancy, for fear it could induce women to drink it by the gallon in the run up to the 40th week in the desperate hope that it will do just that. I'm afraid that, no matter how much you drink, raspberry leaf tea will not encourage that little baby to emerge until he or she is ready. It is, however, full of vitamins and minerals and a great alternative to caffeinated drinks.

effective treatment for back problems, stress, hormonal imbalance and indigestion. One study[11] showed that reflexology is effective for treating a number of different symptoms in pregnancy, as well as speeding up labour. In addition, 89% of the women monitored in the study went on to have a normal delivery.

Like acupuncture, reflexology is also a useful tool for labour induction, and is particularly popular among women who are overdue, because it is thought to stimulate the release of oxytocin, a hormone believed to be essential for starting labour. One of the claims of the practice is that it helps you release endorphins, your body's natural painkillers, which makes it a wonderful therapy for labour.

You can practise basic reflexology at home – perhaps even persuade your partner to have a go after a little training from a practitioner. See page 329 for sources of information on how to find a practitioner in your area.

AROMATHERAPY

I am hugely enthusiastic about essential oils, as they have helped so many women relax during late pregnancy and labour. Lavender is perhaps the most popular because of its calming effects. You can use a couple of drops in your bath, a smear on the heel of your palm before you sleep, or dot it on a hankie and keep it in your handbag to inhale when necessary during the day. Popular choices of oils for pregnancy and labour include geranium and rose, but test them out in advance to make sure you like the smell. Many women burn lavender during labour or use a vaporizer rather than putting the oils directly on their skin, just in case they are sensitive. (For sources of further information on essential oils and aromatherapy, see page 329.)

A CAUTION Like conventional medicine, complementary medicine needs to be used with caution. Certain oils and remedies are not recommended for pregnant women, including: clary sage (although this is useful in labour); clove; jasmine (again, useful in labour); juniper; lemongrass; peppermint (although you can still drink peppermint tea); rosemary; and tea tree oil.

Clary sage is believed to help regulate contractions and so is a popular choice in early labour when things can be a little haphazard, and tea tree can soothe sore places post-labour.

preparing for parenthood

Chances are that you are falling ever more in love with your baby. Perhaps you and your partner have been enjoying the kicks together, pressing back to say 'hello', talking to the baby and discussing every detail of the baby's progress.

Also, you may well have spent some time preparing yourself mentally for parenthood during your pregnancy. But even if you feel as if time has raced by and you haven't properly had time to bond with your baby, don't worry. There is still time to stop, rest, take stock, and carve out some enjoyable quiet moments with your baby.

The baby is now a tangible physical presence alongside you and your partner, and the relationship between the three of you becomes stronger and even more real. Very shortly, you are going to meet this little person and I can suggest ways of making the build up to that moment of birth gentle and enjoyable.

Many women recommend the Hypnobirthing CDs (see page 70) that were not around when I was pregnant, but have become incredibly popular today. There are a few different versions on the market, but essentially these CDs lull you into a state of blissful relaxation in the last weeks of pregnancy and are also fabulous for keeping you relaxed in labour. You can listen to them on your own at any point during the day, while you are having a bath, or leave them on while you fall asleep. Partners enjoy them too – many even claim to sleep better after listening to them.

fears

While this is a magical time, you may also have fears about what life with the new baby will be like. A journey as emotionally intense and varied as pregnancy can bring to light fears, anxieties, unresolved issues and past problems. I strongly recommend that you try to deal with these as they arise. Women who have unlocked deep-held fears and dispelled them have talked about what a difference it has made to them at the moment of birth. Often they felt they were able to enter motherhood refreshed and unburdened.

These may be highly complex childhood issues, they may be new-found fears: what is motherhood going to be like? Can I cope? Can I be a good mother? Will

I love this baby as much as my first child? Try to keep working through any fears and bring them out in the open. If there are subjects you feel you can't discuss with your partner, you can approach your midwife or GP or ask to see a trained counsellor.

It's my belief that all mothers-to-be should have access to a trained counsellor. At some private clinics, such as the Birth Unit at St John and St Elizabeth Hospital in London, this is provided as part of the service.

The Hypnobirthing movement is also a strong proponent of ridding yourself of fears before birth. They have techniques for 'dumping' troubles and fears, and help you learn how to 'let go' during labour. (For sources of Hypnobirthing CDs, see page 329.)

SECOND-TIME MOTHERS

Second-time mothers are usually preoccupied by slightly different concerns. While they have fallen in love with the experience of motherhood and have a real understanding of the miracle inside them, they may wonder how they will ever love anything as much as their first child. They may worry about how they will cope with two. How will their first child respond to the baby? Will the second child be somehow forgotten or neglected? Try to keep working through these fears and to bring them out into the open. With these questions buzzing about in mind, it may be nice to go away for a short break or weekend with just the three of you.

going on holiday

For many women, the last trimester is a time to take stock and reflect. For first-time mothers, it can feel like the end of an era, the end of being 'single', or of being just 'a couple'. It's an end of the leisurely weekend – the lie-ins on Saturday, breakfast and the papers in bed on Sunday.

There are the 'big' questions such as, 'What will it mean to be a parent?' 'What will it mean to be a family (even if that family isn't the conventional Mum, Dad and Baby)?' 'Will I ever have time alone or to just be in a couple again?'

I clearly remember wondering how I would marry two strong instincts within me – that desire to be a strong, independent woman and the seemingly opposing desire to protect and nurture the much-wanted baby inside me. These feelings can be particularly strong for first-time mothers.

For that reason, it can be nice to mark 'the end of an era' with a holiday or weekend break with your partner, or, if you are single, with a friend, or even on your own. I know many women who still remember that last 'freedom' weekend and talk about the 'luxuries' they enjoyed – the walks, the lie-ins, the uninterrupted suppers, the time together, the relaxation. Some even compare it to a sober version of their stag or hen night.

travel

Travel in the third trimester depends on three things:

⊙ how many weeks pregnant you are
⊙ how far you plan to travel
⊙ what mode of transport you want to use.

FLYING

Most airlines will not allow a pregnant woman to fly between 28 and 36 weeks unless she has a letter from her doctor or midwife to say that the pregnancy is healthy. I can't think of any airline that will allow you to fly after 36 weeks.

timing your break

It is generally recommended that you complete your journey by 37 weeks. Even before 37 weeks you should do a bit of research to find out where the nearest doctor, midwife and/or hospital to your destination are based, and don't forget to take your obstetric notes with you. If you go into labour, you may be some distance from the hospital you are booked into. Technically, you are 'full-term' at 37 weeks and could go into labour at anytime, so it's better to play safe.

Also, during the third trimester it's recommended that you have regular antenatal check-ups to ensure that you are not at risk of, for example, pre-eclampsia. If you plan to go away at a time when you are scheduled for an antenatal check-up, ask if you can be checked before you go, so you don't miss seeing your midwife. If you can't be seen at your usual clinic, you can try to organize an antenatal check-up in the area you will be visiting, although this is not always straightforward.

practical preparations for the new arrival

Relaxation is a wonderful way to prepare for the baby's arrival, but there are practical considerations, too. Make sure you have all the nursery essentials you'll need for your baby. Once the nursery is ready, it may seem as if there is nothing else to do but wait. Not so.

BATCH COOKING FOR THE FREEZER

You need to be able to look after yourself once the baby arrives – after all, you'll need to be well fed, calm and rested in order to make sure the baby is well fed, calm and rested.

If you are on maternity leave and you have spare time for making preparations, why not do some batch cooking for the early weeks? Breast-feeding is thirsty and hungry work and you'll be grateful for home-cooked, healthy food that just needs to be reheated. For example, you can freeze home-made stews, pasta sauces, thick soups with plenty of vegetables, fish cakes, pies (such as fish pie, shepherd's pie and cottage pie), pizza dough, stocks and so on.

LOCAL MOTHER-AND-BABY GROUPS

This is also a good time to find out about local groups – in the early weeks you may barely be able to leave the house, but soon enough you will want to meet other mothers with small babies. Your local council can provide a list of all council-run groups in your area. Baby massage groups are good locations for meeting other mums while doing something fun for your baby. Mother-and-baby yoga incorporates exercise and being with your baby. (For sources of information on finding groups in your area, see page 328.)

your hospital bag

Now is a good time to put together the bag you intend to take with you to the hospital and find a safe and accessible spot to keep it. Even if you plan on having a home birth, packing a hospital bag is a good 'just-in-case' measure. If you end up having to go into hospital, you'll be glad you did it. See page 225 for tips on what to put into it.

PRACTICAL ADMINISTRATION

In the postnatal haze, when achieving just one thing in a day is a great accomplishment, you may find simple things like registering your baby's birth or getting a passport an overwhelming challenge. It's worth doing some advance research to find how to do these things.

And it's not just birth certificates. If you are thinking of privately educating your children you may need to get the registration form in as soon as possible after birth, so it's worth making a few calls for application forms now.

ORGANIZING CHILDCARE OR HELP AROUND THE HOUSE

You may find looking after a newborn and keeping up with the household chores – the washing, the shopping, the cooking and cleaning – too much in the early weeks so it's worth thinking about recruiting relatives to help you during this time or, if you can afford it, hiring someone to help you.

Do you think you will need help with the baby? There are a host of options available, from maternity nurses (who can get booked up well in advance) to mother's helpers. You may decide that cleaning help a couple of days a week will cover it, or you may need help with the nights. Use this time to think though the options.

BABY SHOWERS

In the past, relatives and friends would visit the mother and new baby shortly after birth bringing presents for the new baby. Today, there is an increasing fashion for expectant mothers to hold a 'baby shower' in advance of the birth. The baby shower is an American tradition that, like so many things American, has grown in popularity here.

Baby showers are usually an all-female event, organized by a close female friend about three or four weeks before your due date, but there's no reason why you shouldn't throw a baby shower for yourself, have men present, or hold it after the baby has arrived.

The idea is that a group of close friends all get together with presents for the baby. Often, friends will bring clothes, as the chances are that you will have already furnished your nursery – but there's nothing to say you can't hold the shower earlier and ask friends to help you with the essentials.

the final growth spurt

You are now obviously pregnant, and friends and strangers alike will probably comment on your bump and ask when you are due. Also, your baby will be making her presence felt – in the first month of the last trimester (26–32 weeks) you will feel the baby more than ever before. As the trimester goes on, these twists and kicks will be noticeable from the outside. At times, your bump may even shift from its normal shape into awkward, often amusing, forms.

In the last few weeks of this trimester, your baby is concerned mostly with fattening up and will put on an average of 500g (½lb) a week in the last month. The average newborn baby girl weighs 3.5kg (7lbs 8oz) in the UK – that's a big journey from the grain-of-rice-sized embryo you were carrying at six weeks.

WEEKS 28–31: SLOWLY GETTING INTO POSITION

Your baby's head is now in proportion with the rest of his body and, in some cases, he will have already assumed a 'head down' position. All this can still change of course – there is still enough space for some somersaults and twists. Towards the end of this period, however, the baby will feel more confined and will adopt the foetal position, with legs crossed and bent towards his chest.

Your baby has been able to open his eyes for a couple of weeks now and the tear ducts are in place and ready to function. By the end of the 31st week, he is approximately 41cm long and weighs around 1500g (3.3lb), although this can vary hugely. His lungs are the only major organ that are still developing.

Your bump is ever expanding. You so enjoy feeling your baby's movements, and stroking and massaging your bump. You know that you are keeping your baby safe within you, which can be a wonderful feeling. Enjoy eating well, knowing that your baby is getting the best possible nutrition from you.

WEEKS 32–36: FULLY FORMED AND ALMOST READY

All five of your baby's senses are now functioning and she has started to experience dreams – you may even feel little twitches and starts while she is sleeping, and the long stretches when she wakes.

In many cases, the baby will have turned and will now be 'head down' in the pelvis, pressing on the cervix – although in second and subsequent pregnancies this may not happen until labour starts.

Your baby takes deep breaths of water (which is fine as she gets her oxygen from the placenta), and does practice breathing exercises to encourage lung cells to produce more surfactant (a protein that makes the lungs open and close smoothly).

The growth of your baby over the next few weeks is truly astounding. By 36 weeks she is approximately 2000–2500g (4$^1/_2$–5$^1/_2$lb). It can be exciting to feel different parts of her body in your womb. Ask your midwife or obstetrician to help you find the different parts of her body, then you can guide your partner when they are stroking and feeling your baby movements, so that they can share your excitement.

By 36 weeks, your baby is nearly fully grown, usually with her little head down, awaiting her departure date. You'll probably notice her movements more as big stretches rather than the somersaults of previous weeks, as she has less and less space to move. The amniotic fluid is now pooled areas around her body rather than the vast expansive sea at the start of pregnancy, when there was much more water than baby.

WEEKS 37–41: AWARE OF THE WORLD OUTSIDE

Your baby is technically at 'term' from 37 weeks, which means labour from that time on is not considered 'preterm' or premature. First babies, however, are on average born later than their due date. Usually by 37–38 weeks, you will feel a 'drop' as your baby descends into your pelvis. In this position he will be pressing down on your bladder and you might constantly feel the need to pee. His head fits your pelvis tightly and slowly moves down until most of the head is in the pelvis, with very little of it left within your abdomen. Your midwife or obstetrician will see you often to check your baby's growth and movements.

Your baby is now taking up all available space in the uterus and is so large it may feel as if he is deliberately kicking your ribcage. In these final weeks, he can gain as much as a kilogram in weight. He is piling on fat, particularly on his arms and legs, and these fat layers help regulate his temperature. His lungs are now developed and he is drinking amniotic fluid and passing urine in higher volumes. Your baby hiccups because breathing exercises cause amniotic fluid to get into his windpipe.

Hearing is also at its peak and your baby will be turning to hear your voice or any sounds that are familiar or attractive. He will also turn towards – or away from – the light and has definite daily activity cycles. This is a time of much rummaging – he will often have his hands around his face and may even suck his thumb. If you laugh, he will bounce up and down as your abdominal muscles tighten. Often, hiccups are profound at this stage, and you will be able to feel his little jerky movements.

You are now producing antibodies that will protect the baby from diseases after birth.

Your baby is so ready to be born now, the little head bones that move under one another during birth are harder, with little soft parts at the front and back called fontanelles that are useful in determining his position during labour. The vernix that protects his skin from the effects of being constantly wet is almost gone, as has much of the soft, downy hair.

Your baby no longer looks skinny but is rounded. As he kicks, you may start to feel more and more the Braxton Hicks contractions which help give surges of oxygenated blood to your baby as each contraction releases.

Just before birth, your baby's 'practice breathing movements' are very reduced, in preparation for the huge change as air rolls into the lungs at the moment of birth and your baby is out in the world, and in your arms.

As his birthday approaches you will feel an incredible urge to snuggle down, but will also have surges of energy to prepare your nest for your little baby's arrival. Even at this stage, try to hold on tight to the important things – rest, relaxation, positive contemplation, connecting with your baby. Enjoy the last days of having him inside your body, his first home. You will soon meet your gorgeous little baby and hold him in your arms, and see him face-to-face at last.

your antenatal care

Your antenatal appointments will pick up pace in the third trimester and, on average, you will see your midwife or GP once every three weeks from 28 to 37 weeks. From 37 to 40 weeks you will be checked fortnightly and, if you pass your due date, you will have weekly appointments.

antenatal appointments

WHY IS IT IMPORTANT TO SEE THE MIDWIFE SO OFTEN?

Your baby grows rapidly in the third trimester and his or her weight places much strain on your body, and this has associated risks.

You will have another blood test at around 28–32 weeks to check for anaemia. Iron deficiency is responsible for 85% of anaemia in pregnancy, but other reasons for anaemia include folic acid deficiency, Vitamin B12 deficiency, and sickle cell disease. Women with anaemia often look pale and feel exhausted.

TWINS AND MULTIPLES

'Full term' for twins is slightly earlier than with single pregnancies and, if they haven't already, at about 36 weeks your obstetrician will talk you through the different options for your birth. Multiples are always monitored more closely than single pregnancies, so expect to be seen more often. In about 75% of cases, the first twin will be head down. The position of the second twin isn't important at this stage.

Obstetricians recommend that dichorionic (non-identical) twins are delivered by 37–38 weeks, monochorionic (identical) at 36–37 weeks, but if you haven't gone into spontaneous labour by this stage, you will need to weigh up your options. In an uncomplicated scenario you will be given the option to wait for spontaneous labour. Otherwise, you will be given the option of an induction or delivery by Caesarean section.

If you are carrying more than two babies you will automatically be given a Caesarean section.

trusting your body

It is important to let your midwife know if you have any nagging doubts, either about your pregnancy symptoms or the baby. You may not be able to put your finger on the reason for your doubts, but if you explain them, an experienced midwife may be able to pick up something from your 'mother's instinct'.

My policy is always to listen to what a mother says and to check any concerns, just in case. On two occasions in recent years I have seen women who, despite their babies having normal foetal heart rates, have insisted that something was wrong and implored me to do further tests. On both occasions the baby was scanned and subsequently delivered by C-section the same day. Both were as a result of problems with the placenta – there wasn't enough blood supply to the baby – but both babies were fine and healthy once born.

In my experience, a mother's niggling doubt can often be the first sign of something that needs attention so don't hesitate to let your midwife or doctor know. Also, don't be surprised if it ends up being nothing to worry about. There are some quite bizarre side effects of pregnancy. I have known women phone – even attend – the hospital for indigestion, cramps and even haemorrhoids (because of rectal bleeding). In my opinion it's better to be safe, so always speak up.

things you may be concerned about

Tell your midwife, obstetrician or GP immediately if you experience any of the following:

- ⊙ sudden changes in the baby's movements
- ⊙ fears that the bump is not growing as before
- ⊙ very strong period pain-like cramps
- ⊙ a feeling of tenderness when you touch your bump in certain places
- ⊙ sharp pain anywhere on the bump (this can be a sign that the placenta is separating, even if you don't find accompanied signs of bleeding in your underwear).

needs of the mother

The National Institute of Clinical Excellence (NICE) has guidelines on the monitoring of women in the third trimester and these are that 'the needs of each woman should be reassessed at each appointment throughout pregnancy'. This means that each woman should be assessed on her individual needs, regardless of the recommended number of antenatal visits. If you have a concern that you want

needs of the baby

It's not just you and your needs that are monitored in this crucial third trimester. Your baby's needs are greater than ever before, and he or she is more susceptible to hazards.

Make sure you report any bleeding from the vagina early – it may be a sign that your placenta has separated from the wall of the uterus. You should also report urinary or vaginal infections – especially if you have a temperature as it can cause premature labour.

checked or feel that you need to see your midwife more often, you can say so.

Your concerns may be for any number of reasons – not just physical. Perhaps you have concerns about your psychological wellbeing. It's not uncommon for women to arrive at an antenatal appointment in floods of tears. Indeed, sometimes these appointments are the only outlet a woman has and all the trials of her work, home life and relationships come tumbling out.

I certainly believe these issues need to be met by caregivers – women need to be nurtured at this time of tremendous change. I also believe that while an integrated approach is necessary in some pregnancies, the number of health-care professionals a woman sees should be kept to a minimum.

Too many GPs, midwives, doctors and specialists can make a mother-to-be anxious and confused. It can also be traumatic – especially if, say, a mother has been through a bad experience in her first pregnancy and then is forced to repeat the details over and over again to lots of different people.

I also believe that your health-care team need to embrace whoever else you decide to take on the journey to birth with you. That may be your partner, mother, sister, a doula (see page 184) or a therapist. If one of these people is important to a mother in pregnancy, they need to be important to those looking after her, too. In my experience the person – or people – a mother chooses to have with her can have a hugely positive impact on the outcome of the birth.

late scans

I HAD A SCAN AT 20 WEEKS. DO I NEED ANOTHER ONE?

For the vast majority of normal, low-risk births, the answer is no. The job of the midwife or obstetrician looking after you is to examine the position of the baby by hand ensuring, for example, that the baby is not in a breech position, failing to put on weight or surrounded by too much or too little amniotic fluid.

There are exceptions, of course. If, say, you were told you had a low-lying placenta (placenta praevia) at your 20-week scan, you may be scanned again at around 32–34 weeks to ensure it has moved safely out of the way of the cervix.

For high-risk pregnancies, especially with twins (when it is more difficult for the midwife to correctly judge the positions of the babies), you may well be scanned more often.

THE PROS AND CONS OF LATE SCANNING

While the NHS does not routinely scan low-risk normal pregnancies after 20–22 weeks, private obstetricians will often advocate a growth scan at 34–35 weeks. In some cases you may even be sent for regular scans or, if your obstetrician has the equipment in his office, you may be scanned at every antenatal appointment.

In my view the practice of serial scanning is unhelpful in a pregnancy with no complications, mostly because it is unnecessary. It allows the ultrasound diagnosis to replace some of the most important clinical skills of the midwife (and obstetrician). There is a whole range of potential issues that can be diagnosed by simply feeling (palpating) the abdomen. If a scan is used for an examination in place of a pair of practised hands, then the art and science of midwifery and obstetrics begins to be eroded.

It's not just scanning that poses a threat to the field. Caesarean sections are now routinely used for breech deliveries and for twins. This means fewer and fewer midwives and obstetricians are learning the skills needed to deliver breech babies safely, and those skills will, in time, be lost.

I believe that the screening benefits of the scan at 12 and 20–22 weeks is invaluable, but that after that, examinations of low-risk women should be done by assessment. If the midwife believes there is evidence of, say, oligohydramnios (too little amniotic fluid around the baby), a scan can be done to back up those findings.

There are additional arguments about whether excessive scanning can harm the baby and whether boys scanned too frequently are more likely to be left-handed. As I have often said, my rule of thumb is to err on the side of caution and only scan as much as is absolutely necessary in your own case.

WHAT IS THE 3-D SCAN EVERYONE IS TALKING ABOUT?

The 3-D scan is an extraordinary scientific feat in scanning, pioneered by Professor Stuart Campbell, the former Academic Head of the Department of Obstetrics and Gynaecology at King's College Hospital in London. Normal scans show you a 2-D image, usually in black and white. The 3-D image gives a rounded picture of your baby, allowing you to see your baby looking like a baby.

In the case of structural conditions, such as cleft lip or palate, these scans can be very important for determining the extent of abnormality, especially if the baby will require surgery after birth.

In normal pregnancies, however, there is no medical reason to have a 3-D scan. The scan is what I would term 'purely cosmetic'. Because of this, it is not without its critics. Some believe it takes away the mystique of pregnancy and borders on voyeuristic. For those in favour, it is a wonderful way to see their developing child and it helps strengthen the bond with the baby once they can see it in life-like form. The images are not always what people expect, however, and you may not see your baby perfectly. The image 'swims' on the screen and some women have even described it as 'spooky'.

The final point to make about the 3-D scan is that it is expensive – costing approximately £100 (which sometimes includes a video of the experience).

breech babies

Babies that are breech ('bottom down' instead of 'head down') at the beginning of the third trimester still have plenty of time to turn. Approximately 25% of babies are breech before 30 weeks, but that number reduces to 3–4% at term, but some babies will even turn at 41 weeks.

If your baby is still breech by 37 weeks you will have to weigh up your options: you can have a Caesarean section or you can attempt to deliver a breech baby vaginally (see pages 166–7).

In my experience, it is usually the mother that will give the first indication that a baby is breech. Women with breech babies often say things like 'it feels like the baby is kicking on my bladder' or 'there's something so hard under my ribs they feel bruised'. The baby's hiccups are usually felt lower than usual and the heart rate is picked up slightly higher up the abdomen – although this can sometimes be confused with a baby in the occipito posterior position (see page 103).

Midwives also pick up breeches in the course of an abdominal examination – a baby's bottom cannot be moved in the same way as a baby's head. An ultrasound is then used to confirm that the baby is in a breech presentation. That said, 'undiagnosed breech' babies still occur fairly regularly and are usually delivered by emergency Caesarean section.

Sometimes a mother 'just has a feeling' something is not quite as it should be – good old-fashioned female intuition – and, for the most part, doctors and midwives will listen to a mother's concerns. Midwives too can be affected by intuition – I recently saw a woman whose baby was supposed to be head down, but I had a nagging doubt. I referred her to be scanned and my instinct was right: her baby was breech.

There are a number of reasons why your baby may be breech. One obvious example is if you are expecting twins. Another is if you go into labour prematurely and the baby hasn't had time to turn.

Other reasons include, if you have:

- an abnormally shaped pelvis – perhaps from a fracture or it may be something you were born with
- an abnormally shaped uterus
- a 'low-lying' placenta (placenta praevia)
- a history of frequent breech presentations in your family
- a 'lax' uterus or abdomen (one that has been stretched due to reduced muscle tone).

BREECH PRESENTATIONS

There are four types of breech presentation, as shown here.

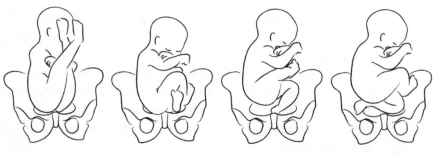

frank or extended   complete or flexed   footling breech   kneeling breech

FRANK OR EXTENDED BREECH 65% of breech babies are in this position, which means the legs are extended and the feet are by the ears. This is the most common breech presentation in first time mothers.

COMPLETE OR FLEXED BREECH This accounts for 25% of breech babies. The baby is cross-legged as with a baby in the head down position. This is considered the best position if you are hoping for a vaginal birth.

FOOTLING BREECH This means the baby is delivered feet first and is rare, but more common with premature babies.

KNEELING BREECH This position is as it sounds, with the baby kneeling. Like footling breech, this presentation is very rare.

'TURNING' A BREECH BABY

If your baby is diagnosed as breech, there are still some courses of action you can take to try to get the baby to turn before having to make a crunch decision about whether to have a vaginal delivery or Caesarean section.

ACUPUNCTURE There is fairly good evidence that acupuncture will help turn a breech baby – some claim as much as a 65% chance at 35 weeks, but there's no knowing how many of these babies would have turned naturally. The procedure is called moxibustion and involves an acupuncturist burning herbs rolled into a cigar shape next to your little toe.

YOGA POSITIONS Crawling on all fours is a popular method for turning a breech baby, as is the 'pelvic tilt' (leaning forward, as you would if you were cleaning the opposite side of the bath). Elkin's manoeuvre – spending 10 minutes in every two hours in the knee-chest position (see page 242) – is also believed to help. Some women have even shone a torch into their vagina to show the baby the exit! However, I have no anecdotal evidence on whether this works.

HYPNOSIS One study[12] has shown hypnosis to be successful for turning a breech. It looked at a group of 100 women who had footling breech babies between 37 and 42 weeks. The women were given relaxation and fear-release hypnosis and separated into two groups. While under hypnosis, the second group was asked why their babies were breech presentation.

getting the baby into a good position

Movement, posture and the position that you sleep in, can all contribute to the baby's final presentation (position in the womb). Malpresentation is one of the most common reasons for a difficult labour. If the baby descends into the pelvis in a tricky position, labour is not only more intense, but longer.

Below are some tips on how to optimize your baby's position in advance of labour (see also the tips on pages 103–4):

⊙ kneel instead of sitting – this will prevent you from slouching backwards
⊙ swim with your tummy down – if your baby is not in the best position, avoid backstroke
⊙ use the 'knee-chest position' (see page 242)
⊙ crawl around the house – this sounds ridiculous, but it does help your baby turn
⊙ use a 'kneeler-rocker' – this little stool devised by Jean Sutton keeps your knees lower than your chest. The combination of that, being upright and rocking helps your baby to rotate. (Look online for sources of the kneeler-rocker.)

If you go into labour and your baby is still not in the ideal position for delivery, don't despair. There are still things you can do to help the baby rotate.

During the first stage:
⊙ walk up and down the stairs
⊙ rock from side to side
⊙ march or tread on the spot
⊙ practise doing figure-of-eight movements with your hips on a birthing ball.

During the second stage:
⊙ get onto all fours
⊙ use a birth stool to help the baby descend (but not for the birth)
⊙ lie down on your left side.

Fortunately, all these positions help you in labour anyway, so there is no harm done if you adopt any of them. In my experience, the vast majority of breech babies do rotate when all these techniques are put into practice.

The study reported that 81% of babies in this hypnosis group moved to a vertex position (head down, chin to chest and curled up in the foetal position) compared to 48% in first group. Although a small study, the results are hugely encouraging. Obviously, hypnosis is most effective on those who embrace it.

EXTERNAL CEPHALIC VERSION (ECV) If natural methods are not turning your baby, you may be offered an ECV, during which your obstetrician or midwife will attempt to turn the baby around using their hands on your abdomen. I should say here that some women find the ECV very uncomfortable, but the success rates are between 50–70% depending on your doctor's record. A few – less than 5% – flip back to breech.

The procedure is usually done after 37 weeks and in the hospital because there is a risk of the waters breaking during the procedure and of labour starting. Other risks are rare, but include placental abruption, uterine rupture and maternal haemorrhage.

Before you are given an ECV you will be scanned by ultrasound to check:

⊙ the baby is still in the breech position
⊙ the baby's weight
⊙ the position of the umbilical cord
⊙ the amount of amniotic fluid around the baby (there needs to be enough
   to support the rotation)
⊙ that the baby's head isn't flipped back (known as 'stargazing').

You will be monitored on a cardiotocograph (CTG) to make sure the baby's heart rate stays stable. The obstetrician will then try to turn your baby by holding his or her head and gently and slowing moving it into a forward somersault. The baby may start to help. The heart rate will be monitored by ultrasound throughout and, if there is any sign of distress, the procedure is stopped.

You will not be eligible for an ECV if:

⊙ you are scheduled for a Caesarean for another reason
⊙ you are expecting twins
⊙ you have experienced bleeding
⊙ you have a low-lying placenta
⊙ your waters have broken

⊙ you have pre-eclampsia

⊙ your baby has a 'hyper-extended' head – where the baby is looking up (or 'stargazing'). Any attempt at ECV in this situation could damage the baby's neck.

ACOUSTIC STIMULATION There is evidence to show that acoustic stimulation may improve ECV success. In one small study, 23 women were divided into two goups – a group of 12 and another of 11. In the group who received acoustic stimulation, 12 out of 12 babies shifted to a lateral position and 11 underwent successful ECV. In the other group, only one of the 11 babies had a successful ECV. These babies were then given acoustic stimulation and a further eight went on to have a successful ECV.

DELIVERING A BREECH BABY

The overwhelming majority of obstetricians in the UK will recommend that you have a Caesarean section delivery if your baby is breech (and cannot be moved), as it is the safest option for the baby. Breech babies can be damaged by a vaginal delivery, and this damage includes bruising to the buttocks, arm injuries (which can lead to arm weakness after delivery), head injury (if the cervix is not fully dilated, or the baby is not chin-to-chest, the head can become trapped in the birth canal after the body has been born).

The Term Breech Trial[13] in 2000 compared nearly 2,100 women randomized into a planned Caesarean delivery group or a planned vaginal delivery group. In the Caesarean group, 17 out of 1,039 babies demonstrated 'serious neonatal morbidity', of which three died. In the planned vaginal delivery group, 52 out of 1,039 showed 'serious neonatal morbidity' – 13 of the 52 died. As the British Medical Journal puts it, the study 'showed a significant increase in perinatal mortality and morbidity (3.4%) with planned vaginal delivery'.[14]

Although this study had a significant impact on UK medical practice – 90% of breech babies are delivered by Caesarean – there are those who argue that it is flawed. They say that, in the planned vaginal delivery group, 22% of the births were not carried out by a trained, skilled practitioner. Those who disagree with the findings argue that the outcome of a breech birth delivered vaginally depends entirely on the skill of the attendant.

Despite the impact of this study, in some cases you still have a choice as to whether you wish to attempt a vaginal birth and some women still prefer to deliver a breech baby naturally. My advice is:

- ⊙ to find out how practised your obstetrician and/or midwives are at delivering breech babies. In my opinion, an obstetrician or midwife who has successfully delivered at number of breech babies shows a good level of expertise
- ⊙ agree a plan with your experienced obstetrician or midwife – this is an example I have used with mothers:
  a I want to go into spontaneous labour
  b I want to be kept calm
  c I don't want an epidural
  d I want to be on all fours or kneeling for the delivery
- ⊙ some women will not agree with this, but I personally prefer to deliver breech babies within mainstream labour wards where obstetric support is immediately available if needed. You can still do this in a birth centre linked to an NHS teaching hospital.

In my experience everything can go fabulously well if the mother is kept relaxed. However, situations can change quickly and the presence of an obstetric, anaesthetic and neonatal team can make a difference in keeping the baby safe.

preparing your mind for birth

Now you are on the home straight of the last trimester, you will really appreciate a few minutes of relaxation in your day. This can be done at any point during the day, in any place.

making a sanctuary

This is a lovely way to prepare for labour. Think about where you want to retreat when labour starts, then turn that place into somewhere you can go to from now to practise your relaxation techniques and visualisations. Many women use their bedrooms, and find a corner to set up a yoga mat and cushions, or use a rocking chair and stool (some women buy them for breastfeeding).

If you are one of those women who don't like to wake sleeping partners if their labours begin at night, your sanctuary may not be in your bedroom. It could involve taking cushions, candles and an incense burner into your

developing your own visualisation

By now, if you have followed the advice on creating your own visualisation (see pages 72 and 128), you will have a fully developed scene, complete with views and elements that ignite your senses. Now return to your special place. See the scene in detail. Let your senses experience everything you have established as part of your visualisation so far. Now think – how does this place make you feel? Joyful, loved, protected, peaceful? Focus on that feeling. Let it rise in your chest and flow through your body until it fills you completely. Is there anyone there with you that makes you feel happy, loved, looked after? Your partner, your child, a good friend or a parent, a relative that died but can be here for you in your mental sanctuary to give you the feelings of love and protection they gave you as a child? Feel that love, feel their arms around you, protecting you and nurturing you. Engulf yourself in all the warm feelings. Remember to breathe deeply as you concentrate on the blissful feelings you are experiencing.

bathroom. It could be your favourite chair in the sitting room. Perhaps you could set up a den in a spare room. Either way, it should be a snuggly spot where you feel completely at ease and can disappear into your head without distraction. You can dim the lighting and play birthing tapes or gentle music, depending on what helps you relax.

visual aids

Using visual aids during labour can be a highly effective way of focusing the mind and shutting out the world in labour, as you breathe, release, relax through contractions. They can also be used as part of a ritual (see page 240) to help you cope. Any picture or object can be used, as long as it makes you happy and calm. One mother I looked after came into hospital with an amaryllis plant.

One of the most successful concepts to come out of The Jentle Midwifery Scheme (see page 11) were The Swirls. These are two pictures that I commissioned from artist Annie Walsh to represent the intensity and beauty of birth. They have been hugely popular as visual aids for labour and women have rated them highly in my antenatal classes. They are now central to my teaching work at Queen Charlotte's Hospital. You can see the swirls and an explanation of their symbolism on my website. See page 329 for details.

I think the reason why so many labouring women have found these images useful is that they represent the birthing process. The first picture symbolizes the wave of a contraction rising, at its peak (the most challenging part), and then receding again – a feeling women can relate to when experiencing the intensity of contractions during the first stage of labour. The second picture represents a mother meeting her baby. I find that women transfer their focus to the second picture as labour progresses (it is especially helpful over the hump of transition and in the pushing 'second stage' of labour).

hypnobirthing

I discovered Hypnobirthing while watching one of my mothers labour. She was not an obvious candidate for self-hypnosis in that she didn't show any preference for 'natural birth' from the outset. However, this was one of those moments in my career when I really learned from a birth. I was astonished at how well she coped in labour – and this was her first birth. Below are her thoughts on this experience and how Hypnobirthing helped her.

CASE STUDY HYPNOBIRTHING

'I am not a hippy or a natural birth person but I thought I would try Hypnobirthing for relaxation. I'd only heard really horrible things about birth and this was my first baby so I wasn't expecting anything. The Hypnobirthing movement say don't listen to anything negative. Believe in yourself and your body: your body won't put you in any pain that you can't cope with. It's all about believing in what women have done for years. I used the CD every night for the last three months of pregnancy and I listened to it every night before I went to sleep.

I was a week late when I had a sudden pain across the lower part of my abdomen. After about 10 minutes it happened again. Then my waters broke. I phoned Jenny and she told me to come in. I got there at 10pm and put the TENS machine on full pelt. My partner James set up the CD player and the oils and I literally just went into a trance. The moment the CD went on I must've been transported to the sleep state that I'd been in every night for the previous three months. I was in complete control of the contractions and remembered what the Hypnobirthing lady had said; that my body wouldn't give me any pain I couldn't cope with.

Hypnobirthing also teaches you to think of a place where you would love to be and at that moment an image came to me: it was a wood across from where I used to live. I was there and I was in control. I've never experienced anything like the effect of this hypnotherapy, but it was very powerful and even though the labour was very intense I was totally relaxed and in control and in this trance. After a bit – I have no recollection of time – Jenny said, "would you like to go into this pool now?" I said "I don't know," because I was actually fine as I was but I didn't know if I would be even better off in the pool, so I ripped off the TENS machine and I tried it. Then James said "You

> "The Hypnobirthing movement say don't listen to anything negative. Believe in yourself and your body: your body won't put you in any pain that you can't cope with. It's all about believing in what women have done for years."

can have gas and air." I didn't know if that would make a difference and Jenny said, "Why don't you try it?" So I did. And the funny thing is that it actually made me lose control. It took me away from where I had been – it knocked me off course. It had actually been better under my own steam and I'd been completely in control, so I went back to nothing. I must've been making some noise because James, who was standing by the pool, then kept saying "you can have an epidural" I just thought, "I'm not listening."

The next moment Jenny said, "Actually you're ready to push. Come out of the pool." So I got out and I sat on a birthing stool and I pushed him out. It had only been eight hours in total – not that I noticed the time. It was absolutely brilliant. It was such an amazing experience. It worked so well for me that Jenny – who had never seen a Hypnobirth before, has since recommended it to loads of women.' KATIE, 34

THINGS TO THINK ABOUT

- ◉ By the third trimester the reality of birth has really taken over and you will be preparing in a number of ways. Not of all these will be in your control – as you will discover when restless nesting takes over. You need to pace yourself – the marathon of labour is not too far away.
- ◉ Your body shape will be weighing you down so this is a great time to work on your mental strength. Remember – your head is stronger than your uterus, no matter how big your uterus is just now!
- ◉ This is the time to think about the things that give you comfort. They will be invaluable in labour. Walk around the house and look out for things that might help you in the grip of labour – do you have a favourite photo, a favourite pillow, a favourite shirt?
- ◉ By now you should be putting the final touches to your Utopia Birth Plan (see pages 175–217). While it's important to stay positive, you can be aware that things don't always go to plan, so factor in a contingency, just in case.
- ◉ If the days turning into weeks are driving you mad, remember 'patience, patience'. Take a walk, go to the cinema, see some friends. Enjoy these last few weeks of peace.
- ◉ Read part two of this book to familiarize yourself with the process of labour and birth.

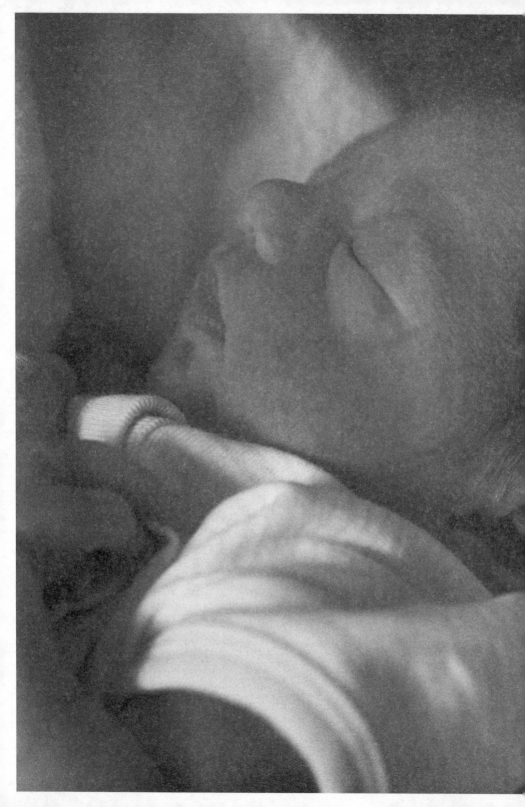

your birth

preparing your birth plan

Your birth plan is your formal declaration to your care providers of what you would like your birth experience to be like. When deciding what to put into your birth plan, aim for your ideal or 'utopia' birth, but also be prepared for the unexpected, which will allow you to keep calm and focused if your labour journey deviates from your plan. If you have a positive spirit, in both mind and body, you will have a positive labour and birth, no matter which way your baby chooses to be born.

your Utopia birth plan

I always recommend to women that they think about how they would like their birth experience to be at points throughout pregnancy. This way, you get a chance to build up your hopes and plans gently, jotting down ideas for your birth plan as you learn more and more about labour and birth. And I also suggest that they aim high – think of how you would like your birth experience to be in an ideal world. You may not get it, but you may well get as close to it as possible. If you build up your knowledge slowly and thoroughly during the first and second trimesters then, during your third trimester, when the idea of birth becomes much more of a reality, you will be ready to write your birth plan.

Many women, first-time mothers in particular, don't know what to expect, either of the physical experience of labour or of the hospital, birthing centre or midwives and obstetricians that attend to them. That is why I take them through the Birth Rehearsal.

the birth rehearsal

The Birth Rehearsal originates from birth preparation classes I held. What struck me was how many women, pregnant for the second and third time, had experienced a traumatic birth, not because of an emergency Caesarean or a dramatic drop in the baby's heart rate, but because of a series of relatively small issues. These, added together, had made for a bad overall experience. In the overwhelming majority of these cases, things could have been different with a bit of good planning.

One of the recurrent themes from those who'd had an unhappy experience was that they did not know their surroundings. They had no idea how the labour ward functioned or who was supposed to be looking after them. Issues such as the birthing pool being in use, or having to wear a hospital gown rather than their own T-shirt, were, in some cases, profoundly upsetting. Also, when 'hospital policy' or 'procedure' dictated that women couldn't do things they had imagined – such as give birth on all fours or in a squatting position – they were left feeling resentful after the experience.

Many women said of their first labours that they remembered seeing a lot of different people whose roles they didn't understand. Some said they didn't know how much freedom they would have to move around, what the machines did, and why they were plugged into them. In the majority of cases, things only went 'wrong' because, somewhere along the line, communication became difficult or confused. I urge you to keep an open mind about your labour journey, plan for the best journey, but also acquire 'coping tools' (such as a knowledge of the medical equipment you may encounter and the epidural process, which you may never need to use, but which may help to keep you calm should you need to use them).

In the following pages I will guide you through a 'virtual walk' of all aspects of labour. By the end of this chapter, you should have an idea of your Utopia Birth Plan and be able to write it up. I discuss all the places you can give birth, the options you have for your birth environment, who you would like to be your birth partner, what you can expect of the hospital staff, and what you can do to make your birth environment as comfortable and comforting as possible. I provide questions that you can ask your care providers so you can discover exactly what is available to you, allowing you to consider how to tailor it to suit your needs.

EXPECTING THE UNEXPECTED

Of course, no good plan is complete without a contingency, as no situation (or very few, at least) is ideal. I like to prepare women to be ready to deviate from their Utopia Plan with as little trauma as possible, by imagining for a few minutes what might happen if things don't run according to the ideal. I like to prepare women for all eventualities and encourage them to embrace any deviation and, of course, to stay positive.

It surprises people to learn that the outcome of a birth can influence a mother long term, and can even shape the way a child is brought up. If a mother is unclear about what is going on around her she may become very frightened or even traumatized. The experience can cloud her entire view of childbirth. I urge you not to skip over the chapter in this part of the book entitled Expecting the Unexpected (pages 264–79) and hope that, in providing you with information about what might happen if things don't go according to plan, I can give you knowledge and information you can mentally refer to when you need it. Knowledge can be a great comfort. Knowing, for example, what the ventouse looks like and what it is used for means that you are far less likely to panic if you see one wheeled into your delivery room.

As women usually attend the Birth Rehearsal with a birth partner, this chapter is also addressed to them. Support is fundamental when labour starts to deviate from the Utopia Plan. Your partner will need to be as calm and reassuring as they can. You need to be able to depend on them to act as a conduit, ensuring that the line of communication between professionals and the labouring mother is open and clear. It is essential that everyone is reading from the same page, especially in an emergency.

Remember that the journey is more important than how the baby comes out. As a midwife I love normal birth, but it is not the most important thing. The main aim is to have a very safe birth – a safe mother and a safe baby. The key message of the Utopia Birth Plan is to be positive. If things go as well for you as you hope, wonderful! But if they don't go to plan, well, you can still be positive because you've prepared yourself for it.

where to give birth

If you are reading this in your first or second trimester, you may think it is too early to start thinking about where you want to give birth. However, if you would like to give birth in a birth centre or want private care, you need to register with them as soon as possible to ensure you get a place.

Today there are many options available in addition to the traditional hospital labour ward. Some hospitals have birth units and there are also private birth centres. There are also private hospital wings. Today an increasing number of women also choose to give birth at home. Recent figures show that 2–3% of women now choose to have their babies at home, and the government is encouraging this practice. Below, I cover the choices available in the UK.

NHS maternity care

As soon as you know you are pregnant it is important to go to your GP and get a referral letter to a hospital so that you have a bed when your baby is due. If you are planning a home birth, you may develop a complication in your pregnancy or need to transfer in labour, so it is still important to get a hospital referral letter.

NHS LABOUR WARD

The vast majority of women in this country give birth on a mainstream NHS labour ward. If you are 'high-risk', you will have access to both obstetricians and midwives and any pain relief available. Mainstream labour wards are fully kitted out with emergency equipment. If you are categorized as 'low-risk' you may be seen exclusively by midwives. You may or may not have met these midwives at your antenatal appointments.

There is an element of 'pot luck' about a birth on a mainstream labour ward. The aim is for each mother to have a designated midwife that attends them during the birth, but if the labour ward is busy, your midwife may also be attending another woman. In the worst-case scenario, you may be having a very fast labour at the busiest time of the year and arrive when all the birthing pools are busy and every midwife appears to be attending someone other than you.

It's much more likely, however, that you will arrive earlier in labour and have time to get to know your midwives and obstetricians. If you have read this book and put in place my suggestions, this scenario could offer you a great birth experience. Use the checklist on pages 190–6 to find out what equipment is on offer and about hospital policies that might have an impact on your birth plan.

Use the checklist on pages 190–6 to find out what equipment is on offer

The advantage of the labour ward is that you will have everything available for any type of birth and access to a specialized team of people who can perform Caesarean sections quickly if necessary. And you will have access to an epidural if you want one. Labour wards are adapting to become more comfortable. At Queen Charlotte's, we have Telemetry, which allows for continuous monitoring of the baby's heart rate without wires, which means a labouring mother can move around.

A quick 'insider's' note – some hospitals will allow you to pay for a private room for one or two nights, even if you have had NHS care up until that point. This gives you both privacy and the chance of rest – at a fraction of the price of a fully private birth.

NHS BIRTH CENTRE

For those who want minimal intervention and minimal pain relief, a birth centre is a great alternative to the traditional labour ward. Birth centres are run by midwives and are for low-risk women undergoing normal births. They have a 'home from home' feel about them, and the midwives tend to support women in their choices for waterbirth, mobility during labour and types of birth positions.

Birth centres are usually stocked with a range of labour equipment including birth balls, stools, mats, birthing pools, rocking chairs and beanbags, as well as the necessary paraphernalia for playing relaxing music or burning aromatherapy oils.

what choices do I have?

HOSPITAL
- NHS hospital (small or big, district or local; NHS teaching hospitals with integrated specialist neonatal services).

BIRTH UNIT OR BIRTH CENTRE
- NHS integrated birth centre (within a hospital), such as that at Imperial NHS Trust and the Birth Unit at Queen Charlotte's Hospital in London.
- NHS separated birth centre where the birth centre is a building completely separate in another location away from hospital.

AT HOME
- With an NHS team of on-call midwives or one-to-one midwifery care.

If a complication arises or you wish to have an epidural for pain relief you will need to be transferred within the hospital or by ambulance to a labour ward in a hospital.

If you opt for a birth centre, use the checklist on pages 190–6 to find out about your local unit.

other types of care

PRIVATE BIRTH UNITS

The majority of private obstetric care is based within and around London. However, there are other private services throughout the country. You can enquire at your local NHS maternity hospital to find out if any obstetricians working there also offer private care.

The obvious advantage of having a private obstetrician is that you will have continuity of care from a person that can perform all types of birth. The disadvantage is that if you wish for a completely natural birth, it might not be the right type of care for you, as not all obstetricians are comfortable with waterbirth, for example.

I have worked with obstetricians who are very relaxed in natural-birth environments, but you will need to check this when discussing your care with them.

Another disadvantage of private obstetric care is the cost, which can be upwards of £10,000.

PRIVATE BIRTH CENTRES OR BIRTH UNITS

At a private birth unit or birth centre you will usually have the choice of obstetrician-led care or midwife-led care. They can, like all private medicine, be expensive – anywhere between £4,000 and £8,000 for midwife-led care – more if you have an obstetrician.

Private birth units, like the NHS equivalent, will also be 'forward-thinking', in that they will adopt the ideas at the forefront of modern midwifery practice such as birthing pools, balls and mats. In most cases you will only be accepted at a birth centre if you are categorized as 'low risk' and your pregnancy goes to full term (37–42 weeks).

The advantage of a private birthing unit is that you will usually be guaranteed one-to-one care with the same midwife (or at least you will be familiar with the midwife or midwives who deliver your baby). They will usually offer fantastic antenatal and postnatal care – including yoga, counselling for all, double beds, baby massage and so on.

The disadvantage is that you will need to be transferred in an emergency. However, many private birth units, such as the one founded by Yehudi Gordon at the St John & St Elizabeth Hospital in London, do have the facilities that allow them to give epidurals and for both emergency and scheduled Caesarean sections.

PRIVATE HOSPITAL

There are a few exclusively private maternity hospitals, of which the most famous is the Portland Hospital, close to Harley Street in London. It is very expensive, upwards of £20,000, for comprehensive care, and it has been renowned as a place for show-business personalities to give birth and be photographed.

Traditionally, the Portland was the preserve of obstetricians and the Caesarean rate was 50% – double that of the rest of the country. They have in recent years introduced a midwifery led package similar to that offered elsewhere.

The advantage of private hospitals or private wings within NHS hospitals, is that you will have access to some of the leading obstetricians in the country. Also, the standard of facilities is usually high, comparable to a hotel. However, private hospitals are very expensive, and on the whole more medicalized in their approach to childbirth.

INDEPENDENT MIDWIFE

You can hire an independent midwife to deliver your baby at home. The most common reason to choose to do this is not being able to access one-to-one midwifery care through local NHS hospitals. Also, some 'high-risk' women (such as those carrying twins or whose babies are breech) would prefer a home birth. I always try to talk very high-risk women into delivering in a hospital for safety reasons.

While I agree that there are some brilliant independent midwives out there, with tens of years of experience, they are not, at this moment, insured in the UK. It's also worth remembering that you will still have to register with your local hospital, even if you are in the care of an independent midwife, and in the event of an emergency, you will still have to go to hospital. Your care will then be taken over by that hospital and their system, and your independent midwife will no longer be able to manage your birth. (See page 327 for sources of information on independent midwives and how to find one.)

home

NHS 'TEAM'

It is a woman's right to choose her place of birth, and in recognition of that fact, many NHS hospitals have put together a team of midwives to deal with home births. While you won't always get one-to-one care, you can usually have your antenatal appointments at home and be in the care of a small team.

An increasing number of women are choosing to give birth at home for a multitude of reasons. Perhaps you had a straightforward birth in hospital the first time and you'd prefer the comfort of home second time around. You may have had a very fast birth first time around and not wish to risk delivering in a car park this time. This may be your dream birth – perhaps many of your friends have had home births.

The advantage of using NHS midwives for a home birth is that they are trained under the auspices of an NHS hospital trust, they are insured, their credentials are up-to-date and they will comply with guidelines set out by NICE. You also have the back up of the hospital in the event that things deviate from your Utopia Plan.

However, depending on what your house is like, you may not be able to enjoy all the benefits available to you at a Birth Centre, such as a birthing pool. (For sources of information, see page 327.)

who to have with you

Your choice of partner through the experience of labour and birth is an important consideration. You need to consider who will best support you through it. It's a good idea to consider this early on in pregnancy because your birth partner should also find out as much as possible about labour and birth, and attend birth preparation classes with you. When we do the birth rehearsal at the hospital I work at, I ask women to bring along their birth partner to the classes.

Your birth partner should be someone who understands your wishes and will speak up for you at times when you are not able to, to comfort you through the pain of contractions and take care of you as you labour.

No first-time mother knows how she will respond to the intensity of contractions. Whereas some women don't need any support and will get on with it regardless of who is present (she may even ask attendants to remain silent), it is much more common for women to go through a period of self-doubt and feeling as if they can't carry on. It is at this stage that a birth partner can play a key role. A simple dose of 'you CAN do it, you're doing BRILLIANTLY, it's going to be fine' is often enough. A labouring mother wants to hear positive talk, even when things deviate from the plan.

options for birth partners

- ⊙ The baby's father
- ⊙ Your mother
- ⊙ Another relative (sister, aunt, etc)
- ⊙ A friend
- ⊙ A doula
- ⊙ The midwives on call that day

THE BEST SUPPORT FOR YOU

Who would support you best through labour? Many women don't hesitate before saying 'the father of my baby' or 'my partner'. Many women in the UK choose their life partners (usually the father) to be their birth partner. For others, it is more complicated. It may sound controversial, but some women do better in labour without their life partners present. I have met women who say they have faltered at the 'self-doubt' hurdle because they did not feel they had their partner's support. For example, a husband may suggest that it is a good time for the labouring woman to have pain relief when all she wants is a little reassurance. Also, some men feel uncomfortable with the process and would prefer not to witness aspects of it. For example, they might prefer to leave the room for all the vaginal examinations and/or for the actual birth, and return immediately afterwards. These men should not be judged for this. Your partner should ask himself the following three questions:

⊙ do you feel shaky at the sight of blood?
⊙ would you be disturbed if you saw your partner empty her bowels?
⊙ are you likely to faint?

A 'yes' answer to any of these questions may mean that he could actually be unhelpful in labour.

It's also important to remember that women need to let go in labour. If a woman is holding back out of embarrassment, her labour might actually slow down. Michel Odent, in his book *Birth Reborn: What Childbirth Should Be*, argues, 'It may not always be best ... for a woman to have her partner there. Certain men have a beneficial presence, while others only slow labour down.

doulas

A doula is an experienced woman (who may or may not have children) who offers practical support to a mother-to-be before, during and after the birth. A doula also offers support to husbands or partners and to other children in the family. Women who want a drug-free birth and an experienced one-to-one companion to see them through that process often opt to have a doula. They can be a great alternative to paying for a one-to-one midwife, and they tend to be a lot cheaper. (See page 329 for sources of information on doulas and on finding an accredited doula.)

In my long experience of doulas, I have found them to be a wonderful support for women in labour. They can act as that woman's 'voice', keeping midwives and doctors clear on her wishes and choices. In instances where husbands find the experience too difficult, they can help women through more intense moments in labour.

However, for that same reason, it is important that your doula and midwife are clear about each other's roles. If a situation arises where your midwife needs to take over, your doula must take a step back.

Sometimes an over-anxious man will get worried and will then tried to hide it by talking too much; his chatter can keep the woman from concentrating on her labour.' Dr Odent continues, 'Men sometimes find it hard to observe, accept and understand a woman's instinctive behaviour during childbirth.'

If your partner is finding it difficult to walk the journey with you, don't get into a battle over it. This is a sensitive issue and must be talked through with him, but his absence can be by mutual agreement, and that doesn't mean there is any problem in your relationship. Think through the alternatives. Could the journey be done with your mother, a sister, an aunt, a friend, or with a doula?

Also remember – you are the one that has to go through labour so, where possible, do not feel pressurized into having someone there that you don't want. Don't be afraid of offending anyone who offers to help. A woman in labour should not be playing hostess to her mother-in-law, for example.

dad's role at the birth

This section is addressed to Dads, whose concerns are often very different to those of the expectant mum, and fathers are often more reluctant to voice their fears in the run up to the birth, either because they are embarrassed or because they don't want to frighten their partner. If you have extreme fears – even if they are quite random – you need to get acquainted with some hard facts so that you can be reassured, and can go on to be a good birth partner for Mum.

I urge you to air your concerns to your partner's midwife. The common concerns I hear from men are:

- ⊙ what if my wife/partner dies in childbirth?
- ⊙ what if we don't get to the hospital in time?
- ⊙ what if there is an emergency with our baby and I can't cope?

Arming yourself with information is the best way to allay extreme fears.

THE FACTS ABOUT THE THINGS YOU FEAR

I often have to tell men that it is very, very unlikely that their wife or partner will die in childbirth. Overall, the UK has one of the lowest rates of maternal mortality in the world.

And while it is certainly the case that some women give birth before arriving at hospital – or even before they have left home – this is unusual for first-time mothers, who are far more likely to have long and more intense labours. If it makes you both feel more confident, talk through emergency plans with your midwife. She will be able to give you advice on 'what to do if the baby comes before the midwife'. In such cases, the mother has usually experienced a painless first stage and is not aware that she is in labour until she feels the urge to push – most women interpret this as a sudden panicky need to poo. If you believe your wife may be in this situation, either you or her should put your hand down there to see if you can feel the baby's head crowning. If you can, dial 999. In the rare event that you have to deliver the baby at home, the emergency services will guide you through what you can do to help your partner deliver the baby over the telephone while they send an ambulance to your aid.

To answer the last hypothetical question above, if there is an emergency with your partner and the baby at the hospital, a team of specialists will be on hand to help and both of you will be talked through the process every step of the way.

FEARS ABOUT A HOME BIRTH

It's very common for people to feel nervous about a mother's wish for a home birth – partners, parents and parents-in-law. In days gone by, home births were normal, but since the Peel Report of 1970, which concluded that hospital was the safest place to give birth, the trend has been to give birth in hospital.

In the last few years, however, there has been an increasing demand for home births and although they still only make up 3% of the total number of births in the UK, that figure is steadily on the rise (15 years ago only 1% of babies were delivered at home).

Home birth is something that needs to be properly thought through and researched by parents (see pages 182 and 203–5 for more information on home birth, and for sources of further information, see page 327). Ideally, both partners need to be signed up to make it a successful and beautiful event. If Dad is not onboard, chances are it's not going to be relaxing, but fraught with anxieties that may affect the mother before or during labour.

Grandparents might even get involved. Perhaps they will be asking Dad, 'What if something goes wrong?' Or saying: 'We don't agree to this plan.' Indeed, those that are ambivalent about home births don't usually come round to the idea until after the event has gone smoothly.

While the place of birth is, fundamentally, the woman's choice, a labouring mother needs support. If you don't feel your partner can provide the support for a home birth, you both need to talk through the options. Would you compromise if she had a natural delivery in a birth centre (if there is one near you), and then went home straight afterwards? Would you be happy for her to have a doula as a labour partner instead of you, but still have the baby at home? Would you prefer her to have a different support network, for example her mother, sister or friends? Would you prefer them to be present at the birth in your place? What are your suggestions and ideas for the birth? Where do you see common ground between Mum's 'perfect birth' and your 'perfect birth'? As with all subjects that cause tensions between couples, a lot of discussion needs to take place well in advance of the birth.

I've had fathers who have been unduly concerned about the following:

⊙ what about the white carpet?
⊙ what if she gives birth in the kitchen?
⊙ what happens if the noise wakes up the neighbours?

Issues like these, thankfully, are relatively easy to resolve, as long as they are voiced in good time. For example, I looked after a mother who kept bringing up the neighbours. I couldn't understand it. She seemed quite calm and surely if this was a legitimate worry she could just give them advanced warning. It turned out it was her husband's fear and it really bothered him. In the end we found a solution: a room where she was least likely to be heard in the street.

FEARS ABOUT A BIRTH-CENTRE BIRTH

As with a home birth, the idea of birth at a birth centre can make some fathers very nervous. They feel that a birth centre is no substitute for a traditional mainstream labour ward. These fears need to be approached in the same way as I outlined above with the home birth. Talk it through and, where possible, find a compromise. Talk it through with the midwives at the birth centre too. Don't be afraid to ask them as many questions as you need in order to find out everything you need to know.

You should also remember that, in the event of an emergency, the birth centre will transfer your partner and baby to the nearest appropriate NHS hospital. (See pages 179–181 for more information on birth at a birth centre.)

your birth environment

In my view, one of the best ways to ensure a woman enjoys the experience of her birth, no matter how much medical assistance she needs, is to create the right environment around her. The National Childbirth Trust (NCT) has conducted two surveys on birth and the results showed that 90% of women polled believed that their environment affected how easy or difficult it was for them to give birth. One in six women said they valued a more 'homely' looking room, offering adjustable lighting, beanbags, mats and the availability of a birthing pool. Of those who said their environment impacted on their labour negatively, 26% said a clinical environment 'hindered' their labour.

While work is being done to improve birth environments on mainstream labour wards, I think the process has a long way to go. That's why I believe women have to be proactive to get what they need. Don't be afraid to ask for things. Don't be afraid to make up a list of things that you want from your birth environment. You do have a say in how your labour is managed, and you do have the right to choose.

your ideal set-up

To state the obvious, the first step towards creating the best environment for your labour and birth is to consider what that environment should be. Below is a list of questions that should help you narrow down your preferences. One of my tips to women is to equip themselves with a 'bag of tools' that will help them stay calm. The more familiar those tools are, the better.

WILL MUSIC HELP YOU?
Try to think about what makes you feel relaxed in your life generally. For example: do you listen to music when you are anxious? Is there any music you have found comforting in your pregnancy? I wouldn't necessarily suggest Elgar or Meatloaf's *Bat Out Of Hell* but it is amazing what some people have to help them relax – I have known women in second stage who want quite loud 'up beat' music to help them through.

If you've been listening to a particular piece of music in pregnancy you may want it in labour, and again to relax with the baby afterwards. I've found that familiarity can be a great comfort to women who are feeling a little stressed. In this way a familiar piece of music can be a wonderful tool. Perhaps you prefer the noise of the everyday to make you feel grounded. I know three women who gave birth listening to BBC Radio Four. Or maybe it would be the lulling tones of the Hypnobirthing affirmations that would reassure you.

Or perhaps you prefer complete silence.

DO YOU FIND WARM WATER RELAXING?
This is an interesting one because some women think they will find it relaxing but, in the event, they don't use the bath or birthing pool. That said, the power of water is a tremendous prop for some women. Often just watching the surface of the water, or putting a hand in and feeling it against your skin, can be very soothing.

DO YOU THINK YOU'LL WANT TO WALK AROUND IN LABOUR, OR RETREAT INTO A CORNER AND BE STILL?
In my experience, women find repetition very useful in labour – whether it is returning to a certain place in a room for support, repeating a sound or mantra, or focusing on a certain spot to help them concentrate. I call this 'the rituals' of labour.

respecting a mother's wishes

This is an issue that is often overlooked in all the arguments over how birth is managed. Some very high-risk women feel that they are being talked over by those who wish to merely discuss the clinical procedure of their birth, and don't take into account what will make the mother feel comfortable or nurtured.

In 2007, the Safer Childbirth report reasserted the importance of a mother's wishes and her involvement in the decision-making. This is the point of a birth plan, and to make this work, women need to understand what their choices are and what they mean in terms of risk. They then need to be supported, whatever their decision.

DO YOU THINK AROMATHERAPY OILS WILL BE COMFORTING?

As midwives in general are not trained in aromatherapy, you need to bring your own oils with you. Do some research into their properties and into the smells that you like (see left). I usually suggest to women that they heat their oils in the room rather than rubbing them onto the skin, but you can dab lavender oil onto the heel of the palm and then rub your hands together and inhale it or put it on a hanky. If you bring a burner, make sure it is electrical as live flames can't be used.

aromatherapy oils for labour

Popular choices are:

- ⊙ lavender – both relaxing and balancing, but also has healing properties
- ⊙ rose and frankincense – relieve fear and anxiety, promote relaxation
- ⊙ clary sage and jasmine – stimulate and strengthen contractions.

ARE THERE ANY PICTURES THAT MIGHT HELP YOU IN LABOUR?

We've discussed photographs that might help visualisations such as mountains or waves crashing against the shore. We've also touched on The Swirls, which many women find a huge help (see page 169). Some women find encouragement from looking at photographs of their other children as babies. Perhaps a scan photo will spur you on.

The illustrations on pages 258–9 may help you visualise your baby moving down the birth canal. It will also help you imagine what is going on inside. Looking at pictures like this is very helpful as you near second stage. It is nearly always an intense moment and many women find that focusing on the baby's head coming down, and the idea that you will shortly meet this tiny being, is the best way to get through it.

questions to ask your care providers

Now you've thought about the elements you can bring to birth that may help you feel relaxed, you need to adapt them to the environment that is on offer at the place where you plan to give birth. To help prompt you, I'm going to walk you through some of the options so you can ask your care providers what is available at your hospital or birthing centre. But I also offer tips on how to adapt seemingly unfriendly surroundings to your advantage and help create your ideal birth environment.

IS DIMMED LIGHTING AVAILABLE?

Turning down all the lights in the room is one of the most important ways of creating the right environment in labour. It closes the room down; even quite a large room can feel smaller. It can also help women go 'into themselves' – a basic part of coping in a labour with no pain relief. Bright lights can be very distracting. Most of the women I look after choose dim lighting while in labour. One simple way of doing this is by placing an angle-poise or examination light against a wall to reduce the glare, then switching the overhead light off. Ask if the hospital can be flexible with the lighting and if they mind if you adapt the lighting to make a room darker?

WILL I HAVE TO MOVE ROOMS FOR DELIVERY?

If so, what is on offer in the delivery room? This is an important question because, if you have laboured alone in a dark room for several hours and then suddenly have to move to a brightly lit suite full of people in order to give birth,

'bring your own'

If you find your local hospital too clinical, adapt the environment with a bit of 'bring your own'. For example:

⊙ bring your own pillow – especially useful if you don't like the scratchy starched NHS pillow cases
⊙ if no birthing ball is available, bring one (for retailers who supply them, see page 329)
⊙ bring your own CDs and something to play them on
⊙ bring your own aromatherapy oils

and a burner. I think the electrical diffusers work best. They are made of porcelain and you place the oil on top of a hot plate to burn it. Obviously make sure you like the smell in advance of using it – women are very sensitive to smells in labour, and burn only two at a time
⊙ bring your own homeopathic remedies – Bach rescue remedy is good for transition, arnica is good for bruising.

the change of environment can be startling and distracting. (This will obviously happen in an emergency situation.) The National Childbirth Trust's audit on labour and environment (published in September 2005) showed that even very simple changes to a birthing environment could make a difference to the outcome of a labour.

DO THE LABOUR ROOMS HAVE ENSUITE BATHROOMS?
Many hospital labour rooms do have ensuite bathrooms but don't assume they do. If yours doesn't, you may want to find out how far away the toilets are from the labour rooms. It is not uncommon for women to strip during labour because they feel suddenly very hot. If the bathroom is across a public corridor you need to work out in advance what you can put on to get there. A dressing gown would be useful in such a scenario.

DO THEY HAVE BIRTH BALLS?
If so, are these on offer for everyone? If not, can you bring your own? (You can use one of the big silver balls they use in gyms, which are available from Argos for around £10.) Balls are marvellous for sitting on, doing figure-of-eight exercises, or for leaning over. They are usually available, but you may like to bring your own as different people suit different sizes. And if you're not using it, it can always be something for your labour partner to sit on.

DO THEY HAVE OTHER EQUIPMENT AVAILABLE?
Do they have rocking chairs, matresses or beanbags? I find beanbags are quite an individual prop so it's probably a good idea to try them out beforehand to see how it feels to lie over or kneel on. Some women find them very comfortable, some don't. In my experience, they are best used propped up against a wall in order to keep them bulked up – when they are soft they don't give enough support.

I find they are most useful during the second stage, when you can lie over them while kneeling on a mat, in a fairly upright position, which helps the baby come down the birth canal.

CAN I DELIVER MY BABY ON THE BIRTH MAT?
A birth mat can give you more flexibility in terms of the position you give birth in. Many women like the all-fours position or squatting in a supported position

with their partner, and in these positions, birth mats are useful as something soft to fall on.

ARE BIRTH STOOLS AVAILABLE?

If so, try them out. They can be very useful in labour, particularly during the second stage with women who have had an epidural as it helps them to feel the pressure in their bottom (although not for delivery if you have had an epidural, as the tearing can be significant).

The stool allows you to get this pressure into the bottom area and to feel the baby coming down. It therefore helps you focus on the spot you need to push down into – or breathe down onto, if you are doing the Hypnobirthing method. If birth stools are not available, you can use the loo as a temporary birthing stool in labour (although not, obviously, for delivery).

ARE BIRTH POOLS AVAILABLE?

Government guidelines recommend one pool for every 1,000 births. However, many hospitals, birth centres, and even some of London's most famous private hospitals, do not have them.

If one is available, ask to have a go when you are on a tour of the labour ward. Put your knees in the bottom and try it out with some pillows. Think about which position you might be in during labour – you could be kneeling or lying down. Remember that, when the pool is full of water, you'll need to keep your bottom below the surface of the water. Move around the space to get a feel for it.

It's also worth remembering that while birthing pools are now an essential part of NHS scenery, not all maternity staff will be qualified to oversee a birth in a pool. Where they are found, they can also be in high demand. I think it's very important not to set your heart on the pool if you believe there is any chance it may be in use.

If you don't have the option of a pool, ask for a bath. You can't deliver your baby in it, but you can get that wonderful sense of the warm water over you. Try the shower on your back too. This can be a great compromise on losing out on the pool. I can think of many cases where women have been so happy with the situation, even when they have had to compromise, because they had been prepared and had a positive attitude towards it. Think positively about possible solutions to any problems.

Questions to ask your hospital or birth centre might be:

⊙ how many pools do you have?
⊙ what are my chances of using the pool?
⊙ if the pools are full, can I have a bathroom with a shower on my back?

IS THERE A CD PLAYER OR SHOULD I BRING MY OWN?

What is the hospital or birth centre policy towards you bringing your own music?

CAN I MOVE AROUND?

Find out if it will be possible to move around if you need to. Ask: can I get off the bed? Can I lie on the floor? Can I walk around the ward? If you know you're a walker, it might be worth testing how much space you may have.

WHAT IS THE HOSPITAL POLICY ON MONITORING?

Does your hospital have the latest high-tech equipment such as telemetry (remote monitoring)? This might be an important question for high-risk mothers who need constant monitoring, but would like a low-tech experience and a little 'normality' in their birth experience. If there's no telemetry, can you walk the length of the wires? Ask to see the CTG machine and the tocograph.

WHAT IS THE HOSPITAL'S ATTITUDE TO PAIN RELIEF?

Entonox (gas and air) is usually available, even in home births. On a visit to the labour ward you can ask to hold the machine to familiarize yourself with it. Knowing the equipment on a ward can make any changes to your birth plan much easier to cope with.

At some birth units it is not possible to have an epidural; elsewhere it's not encouraged, so if you think you might want one, you'll need to find out if one is available to you. At the other end of the scale are private hospitals, where the epidural rate can be as high as 80–90% or more (and where you may be asked to wear a gown with an open back, even if you don't want an epidural).

Some women who intend to have a natural birth do, in the event, request an epidural. If your intention is to have a natural birth, it is worth finding out if an epidural is available at your intended place of birth, should you change your mind when it comes to the big day.

hospital staff and their hierarchy

DOCTORS
Doctors are required to do regular training to maintain their registration.

CONSULTANT The top grade for obstetricians. Usually a man, but there are an increasing number of female obstetricians. They can deal with any labour emergency and know how to pull other members of the team together if needed. He or she is very senior and is a member of the Royal College of Obstetrics and Gynaecology (RCOB).

SENIOR REGISTRAR A senior grade (very experienced) obstetrician. This is someone – like the registrar – who delivers babies all the time.

REGISTRAR A middle-grade level in the obstetric team.

SENIOR HOUSE OFFICER A junior-grade level in the obstetric team.

ANAESTHETISTS Specialists in field of pain relief, including epidurals and general anaesthetics.

NEONATOLOGISTS Hospital-based paediatricians who specialize in newborns who require special medical care.

MIDWIFERY STAFF
It is more than likely that a midwife will be the person who will see you through labour and, in the majority of cases, that will be all you need. However, it is comforting to know that if anything should become abnormal, she or he will refer you to a doctor.

DIRECTOR OF MIDWIFERY The most senior midwifery position in the maternity service.

HEAD MIDWIFE A senior midwife in the hospital/community.

SENIOR MIDWIFE A 'level seven' midwife. She or he coordinates all the mothers in the area, prioritizes and ensures that the doctors are aware of any problems.

MIDWIVES These are 'level six' midwives who are experienced and registered with a statutory body such as the English National Board of Nursing and Midwifery. Every year they have to state to a central register their intention to practise as a midwife.

Everyone employed by an NHS Trust is covered under vicarious liability insurance for both hospital and home births.

what should I expect of the hospital staff?

Most midwives work in shifts. The midwife you see when you arrive may not be the one present when you give birth. Try to utilize your birth partner to the fullest and have a good idea what will help you in the hours that you are labouring without any hospital professionals.

Another area that is worth finding out about is the hospital personnel that you will encounter while you are in labour – who will be popping in and out of your room and who the hospital will have present at your birth. You could ask the hospital staff the following questions:

- ☉ how many people are allowed in the delivery room?
- ☉ what is the maximum number of attendants if my birth is straightforward and low risk?
- ☉ what about if you have any concerns?
- ☉ will there be students or trainees?
- ☉ what is the staffing ratio at this hospital?
- ☉ will I be left without a midwife at any point? If so, for how long?

types of birth

Some women don't have much choice in the type of birth they can have. For various reasons, some have to have a Caesarean section; others may be limited by the facilities on offer. But for most low-risk and many high-risk mothers, there are a number of options available that should be explored. This section runs through the different types of birth you can have. Read the notes on each one, so you will be that much more prepared for sudden necessary changes of plan.

natural birth

Many women say to me, 'I want a natural birth.' What do they mean?[15] The dictionary defines it as 'a method of childbirth in which medical intervention is minimized and the mother often practises relaxation and breathing techniques to control pain and ease delivery.'

It could be (and it has often been) argued that a truly natural birth requires no intervention whatsoever. That means there would be no 'natural' inductions, such as cervical sweeps, acupuncture or reflexology, because how natural can an induction be? There would certainly be no artificial rupture of the membranes (waters), and even a manual rotation of the baby's head in labour is questionable because it is, in effect, interference.

In its simplest, stripped-back form, a truly natural birth would have to be a spontaneous vaginal birth at home with minimum assistance – and given that accounts for only a tiny fraction of births in the UK today, I think we can safely assume that is not what the vast majority of women are asking for.

In both obstetric and midwifery circles, the debate continues as to what actually constitutes a 'natural birth'. However, from my own corner of the field of midwifery, I see women who are reacting against the rising rates of Caesarean section and heavily 'medicalized' births. I see women who are very high-risk who feel nervous about the prospect of ending up with quite a serious operation at the end of their pregnancy. When they ask for something 'natural', they want to get as close as possible to an experience where they can feel involved and in control of their birth.

So when women say to me, 'I want a natural birth', I understand them to mean that they would like to try for an experience with as many 'natural' or 'normal' elements as possible. I try to help them achieve that.

CAN I BE 'HIGH-RISK' AND STILL ENJOY A NATURAL BIRTH?

The short answer is yes. When planning a birth, even with the most complicated pregnancy, I try to get mothers to think of the little things that would make their experience a little more 'natural' or 'normal'. I call this 'normalizing the abnormal'. For example, one woman said of her labour, 'My husband and I hugged throughout labour. The lights were down and we shared special moments.' An outsider would not immediately guess that was a quote from a mother who was high-risk and thus heavily monitored.

Instead of setting out from a position of what a high-risk woman cannot have, I prefer to start with all the things she can have. For example, you can have a massage, dim lighting, music, snuggly bits (items from home that make you feel more secure during labour), beanbags and mats. You can walk around, sit in a rocking chair, do 'labour dancing' (movements that ease the pain of contractions), hug your partner and get up and go to the loo. On hearing this, most women immediately feel much more positive about their births. The 'can't' bits can be fitted in around the 'natural' bits. Yes there will be compromises, but don't be afraid to question the choices you are offered.

Below are some examples of areas you could question and how.

- ☉ If you don't immediately plan to have an epidural but are told you have to wear a gown with an open back, ask, 'Why? I haven't decided on an epidural yet and I am more comfortable in my own clothes.'
- ☉ If you are told you can't wear your own pyjama top in theatre, ask, 'Why not? The top end of my body is not a sterile field.'
- ☉ If you are told you have to be on a bed for a premature birth, ask, 'Why? If the emergency measures are in place, I can be on a mat on the floor.'
- ☉ If you are told you can't have a waterbirth after an induction, you can ask, 'If there is continuous monitoring in place, why not?'
- ☉ If you are told you can't see your baby come out during a Caesarean, ask, 'Why can't you drop the screen and let me watch?'

'It was meant to be a "difficult" pregnancy because I've got a liver disorder that means when I am pregnant I get severe obstetric cholestasis, which was diagnosed during my pregnancy with my son George. I went into spontaneous labour at 30 weeks and he was in the Intensive Care Unit for two months. When I got pregnant with Annabel, my doctor, Catherine Williamson, an obstetric medicine specialist, expected that I would have OC again.

It started in the first trimester, at about eight weeks. I was a bit apprehensive as it had been so bad with my first pregnancy, but I started the medication and I had Jenny and Valda as my midwives, which was very comforting. So as the pregnancy went on, I didn't feel high-risk at all. Other than a bit of discomfort at night, I began to quite enjoy it, which was very different from the last time, which I hated.

By 33 weeks my condition was worsening and the decision was made to deliver the baby. The whole team – Cath, Jenny, Valda and a counsellor called Jenny Chambers who had also suffered from OC – were all there for support.

George's birth had been very controlled. I think, looking back, that everyone was quite worried during his birth. I was on the bed and I wasn't allowed to move and it made me nervous. It was like I was chained to the bed, I felt like a prisoner really. With Annabel's birth it was completely different.

'I had music and incense and a natural birth – it was amazing. I got to hold her straight away.'

It was as relaxed as it could be. I was in a nice room with twinkling lights and I didn't have to stay attached to the bed – I was allowed to walk around. After the induction, I even went out for a walk with my husband Jamie and we sat on a patch of green near to the hospital. It was really nice.

Because of the support of the two Jennys it was actually a fantastic experience. After about 12 hours Jenny (Smith) broke my waters to speed things up. She and Jenny Chambers were really supportive and it was so relaxed. Jamie felt the support of the team was fantastic because at any time that he felt overwhelmed they took over.

I had music and incense and a natural birth – it was amazing. Annabel was born just after midnight and weighed 4lb 15oz. To me she looked enormous because my son was only 3lb 3oz. Looking back she was just a dot.'
RACHEL, 23

waterbirth

Waterbirth has become increasingly popular in the UK and is now an accepted norm and many women hop into the bath in the early stages of labour at home. Water has been shown to be hugely beneficial in many ways – as a form of pain relief, for relaxation, to help labour progress and to avoid unnecessary intervention. It doesn't even need to be a tub full of water; back labour pain can be greatly relieved by a powerful showerhead trained on the area of pain.

Approximately 295 maternity units in the UK have a birthing pool, 20 of them have more than one.[16] It is now recommended that there should be one birthing pool per 1,000 births.

If your labour is progressing normally, there is no reason why you shouldn't be allowed access to a birthing pool, if one is available. Using the pool as a form of pain relief for the first stage, and actually delivering the baby in the pool are two quite different propositions. If you want to actually give birth under water, it's worth thinking it through beforehand.

IS IT FOR YOU?

Waterbirth is magical and beautiful. It is, however, not for everyone. You need to be aware of the pros and cons. Think about whether you find water helpful for pain or calming in your everyday life. Are you someone who runs a bath to help with period pain? Is a bath a place where you relax? How do you feel about water? Are you completely comfortable with water?

If you feel uncertain, then it is probably not right for you. In my experience women who want waterbirths know they want them. If you have established that it is right for you, the next thing you need to check is whether there are midwives available who are qualified to deliver babies in the birthing pool.

AN IDEAL WATERBIRTH

In an ideal waterbirth, you want to get into the pool once you are around 5cm dilated. You need to feel calm, with the endorphins flowing. The use of dim lighting makes the experience feel more private.

Currently, there is no real consensus on what temperature the pool should be. I usually keep it at about 37°C. There is a sense of being separate once you are in the pool – your have your own little moat around you which guarantees private space. The midwife and caregivers are distanced from you and, although they can reach you to monitor the baby, they don't get in with you. I have had women who have invited their partner in wearing underwear, but it's not very common.

You do need to be in a suitable position to have the baby's heart rate checked with an underwater Doppler – around once every 15 minutes in the first stage, and after every contraction in the second stage.

When it comes to delivering in the pool itself, you need to fully appreciate that for one contraction, the baby's head will be out and underwater, but the baby's body will still be inside you. This can be daunting. Midwives often don't like to touch the baby while he or she is underwater in case it stimulates the baby to take a breath, but this can be wonderful for the mother, who can get to be the first person to hold her baby. Once the baby's body is born, he or she can then be lifted straight up to you out of the water.

It's important to be well supported straight after you've had the baby, as there's a relaxing moment when all the endorphins flood in and you may flop. The pool is a wonderful place to be at that point. You'll need to make sure the baby's head remains above the surface of the water at this point. Sometimes the wave of relaxing endorphins can make women feel woozy. Your partner should help you hold the baby firmly, and the midwife may lower the water level.

WHEN THE PLAN MIGHT CHANGE

A waterbirth stops being suitable if you are so uncomfortable in labour that you find yourself thrashing about. In this case you need to come out and try something else – perhaps pacing the floor. Some women need stronger pain relief.

Deep water can slow labour down and long-term immersion is not thought to be ideal for babies. If your labour is taking longer than anticipated you may need to come out. Another reason you may need to leave the pool is if you have diarrhoea, or if there are any changes to the baby's heart rate. Once the baby's head is born, the body needs come with the next contraction. If not, I ask the mother to get out to check whether the shoulders are stuck or if there are any loops of cord around the baby's neck.

If at any point the midwife does ask you to leave the pool, you need to do so quickly. (I practise this with my waterbirth mothers in the birth rehearsal.) This also applies after the baby is born and if any bleeding occurs, as you may need a syntometrine injection to speed up the delivery of the placenta.

'I've got three boys, James, Thomas and William. James had been a planned home birth, but it was not a good experience. I had two wonderful midwives but unfortunately James didn't progress very well. One of the midwives had already been on a shift and she had to go. A new one was called to help the fantastic male midwife, but she didn't participate or support, she just sat on my birth ball in the corner. This is the point at which (I realise in retrospect)

> 'It was amazing. I was really confident that the baby was going to be happy about this because he had been in water for nine months. I love water anyway and it just felt very natural to me.'

I went into transition and felt like I couldn't go on. Instead of the male midwife being able to say, "Maybe we need to give it a little longer and see what happens," the midwife on the birth ball was saying, "Let's just go in." She wasn't pro-home birth.

So I was taken straight into emergency and I felt I had no one to talk to. My contractions were very strong but the surgeon just carried on talking through them, not even giving me a break to breathe. Next thing I knew I had been signed up to a Caesarean section without wanting or necessarily needing one. Once you are in the system you are in the hands of the surgeons and you are locked on that route where people want to interfere. I didn't feel experienced enough to put my foot down and say, "No that's not what I want."

I came away feeling very disappointed, but also very annoyed that I'd had this operation that I felt I didn't need, and because of it, next time around I might have to have a Caesarean section.

When I was pregnant again, I met Jenny. She very kindly said she would consider me for a home birth even though it would be a VBAC at home, but then the pregnancy became complicated and it was clear that I would be going to hospital. My husband and I looked into the statistics on VBACs. We knew Jenny had a lot of experience and we trusted her. If at any point you think there is going to be a problem, you need to be able to trust the person you are with.

Fortunately, I went into natural labour, but again it was difficult. I'd read all these idyllic stories about the endorphins kicking in and natural labour being wonderful but I don't remember seeing any saying, "It's bloody painful, it's bloody awful and in fact you can feel really terrible afterwards." I tore and to me it was really painful.

William, on the other hand, was a straightforward pregnancy. I knew my body by the time I had William. I felt really confident that I knew what I was doing. It was fantastic. I went into labour and we went to the delivery room, I was confident enough to leave it a bit later before going in and time went a bit quicker. I got into the birthing pool and stayed there all the way through. I didn't know until afterwards that it is very unusual having had a Caesarean to have a baby underwater. It was amazing. I was really confident that the baby was going to be happy about this because he had been in water for nine months. I love water anyway and it felt very natural to me. My husband said, "It was a little bit more elegant than lumbering around on a beanbag."

Jenny was diligent in ensuring that the medical side of things was in place. The best thing about it was that it was very cathartic and redeeming because, although the next day I did feel awful and my body was weak and painful, it didn't get me down; I was confident.

Afterwards we had the double bedroom and how much more natural to have that room and all be together as a family. I feel amazingly privileged to have been able to have the experience I had with Jenny in that I had choices. It seems so unfair that so many other women can't have midwives who support them in something like this.' DIANE, 41

HIGH-RISK WOMEN AND WATERBIRTH

High-risk women are not excluded from having waterbirths – indeed some women have been adamant that they want one. I have helped look after women who, for example, are having a vaginal birth after a Caesarean section, or who have been induced. In these cases, we have used underwater telemetry to monitor the foetal heart rate at all times.

home birth

Home birth has enjoyed a recent surge in popularity and, today, as many as 3% of women give birth at home. To be eligible for a home birth with the NHS, however, you need to be low-risk and to have enjoyed a straightforward pregnancy. As with a birth-centre birth, you cannot have an epidural, but you can have gas and air.

Your midwife needs to come to your home in advance of the birth to see if it is a suitable environment. She (or he) will advise you on what you need for the birth – I usually recommend an old duvet (to kneel on and to wrap around you if you get cold) and lots of towels that you can throw away afterwards.

If you want to have a waterbirth at home, you need a room that is big enough to hold a pool and where the floors are strong enough to support it. The pool also needs to be filled from a tap, so one needs to be at hand. You also need to think about how you are going to drain the pool afterwards.

Home births can be wonderfully relaxing; you are in your own environment, you can burn candles, dim lights, have aromatherapy in your bath, and eat your own home-made food during labour. They are also great for partners and other children – the family can all get into bed together after the baby is born.

At the first sign of an emergency, however, your NHS midwife will insist on 'blue lights' (an ambulance). I make sure that all my home birth mums understand this and, on the rare occasions when this has happened, we managed to keep to a 'utopia contingency plan' in place.

CASE STUDY **HOME BIRTH**

'I am not particularly political about childbirth – I think women should do what they feel most comfortable with. I have quite a broad cross-section of friends and so I know women who have gone for elective Caesareans as well as home births.

I was listening to one friend describe her home birth and I thought it sounded really calm so I decided I would look into it. I did a lot of research – partly for myself, partly so that I could respond to all the people who questioned my judgement – and a lot of preparation. I took Hypnobirthing classes with the attitude that if it helped, well great, and decided to be very positive about the birth.

Towards the end of my pregnancy I was taken aback at how many people gave their opinion on my choice. I remember one woman telling me how mad she thought I was and asking why I hadn't got a consultant obstetrician. A lot of people wanted to focus on the mess, asking if I was worried about my floor or carpets. I can't imagine people feeling so free to comment on any other type of birth. Anyway, I stuck with feeling positive and fudged enquiries into where I was giving birth.

I had a long run up to labour, with a few weeks of strong practice contractions. In fact, the night I actually went into labour I kept going back to sleep between contractions thinking it was a false alarm. I was still asking if it was for real when the midwife arrived and I was about 8cm dilated.

It was very calming to be at home. There was no underlying panic about when to leave and go to hospital. I could eat, sleep, use my own bath, light candles and generally feel very quiet and relaxed. I would say that the contractions were very intense, but they never really hurt. Every time I felt a wave come on, I concentrated on relaxing into it, making sure my shoulders were low and my jaw was "softened".

> 'It was very calming to be at home. There was no underlying panic about when to leave and go to hospital. I could eat, sleep, use my own bath, light candles and generally feel very quiet and relaxed.'

At transition, I asked my husband to get me a cup of very sweet tea and went off alone to lie on my bed and listen to the Hypnobirthing CD. When it was time to push, I knelt down and tried to focus my breathing down rather than out. The actual point of birth was the only moment that I thought about gas and air and the thought was, "I guess it's a bit late to ask for that gas cylinder now."

Ten minutes later I was in my own bed with the baby in my arms and a big plate of toast. It was really idyllic. I always think it's strange when people say, "you're brave". It wasn't done for bravery. It was just a much nicer experience.'

CLARE, 29

elective Caesarean section

If this is your first pregnancy, then the most likely reason you will be considering Caesarean, unless the circumstances of your pregnancy require you to have one, is that you have fears about labour and birth. Tocophobia is the term for an extreme fear of labour. If this describes how you feel, speak to your obstetrician as early in your pregnancy as possible, so that specialist help can be given to you, in terms of both psychological and physical support.

If this is a subsequent pregnancy, you may be considering a C-section because you had one previously. Some women don't wish to take on the risks associated with a vaginal birth after C-section (VBAC), such as a 1 in 3 chance of an emergency Caesarean, and a 1 in 200 chance of uterine rupture (see pages 220–1). But it is important to note that you do have a reasonably good chance of achieving a successful vaginal birth after a C-section (see pages 218–21).

Also, if you do achieve a vaginal birth following a Caesarean, your chances of another vaginal birth after that are much higher, and your risk of uterine rupture also reduces. If, however, you do opt for a second Caesarean, it will be obstetrically recommended that you have further Caesareans as the risk of rupture increases. If you go beyond two Caesareans, surgery is more difficult and the risk of haemorrhage is increased.

CASE STUDY **ELECTIVE C-SECTION**

'I was keen to deliver my first child "naturally". I met Jenny and felt she was so experienced, relaxed and upbeat that she would be the perfect person to counter my rather anxious disposition and help me through my fears. All went well with the pregnancy and I had devised a birth plan – I was hoping to have a waterbirth, using the birth pool for pain relief as far as possible. At about 34 weeks, my baby was still in breech position. I was given a couple of options for turning the baby: trying out exercises or going for external cephalic version (where the doctors manually turn the baby from the outside of the abdomen). I didn't want to have the external cephalic version as I had a strong family history of breech births (my mother had three out of four breech presentation babies and my grandmother had three out of three) and I thought that perhaps there was a good reason my baby was in this position, so manipulating it into another one felt counterintuitive. The exercises didn't work in my case, so elective C-section was my safest option for delivery. I was concerned about a C-section because it is after all a pretty

'My wonderful baby snuggled into my neck, a feeling I will never forget. We were given the skin-to-skin time, which was so important to me. Within 30 minutes of his being born, Jenny helped me position my son to my breast and he fed greedily.'

major operation and I had really wanted the moment of skin-to-skin with my baby immediately after delivery especially as I thought this would help with breastfeeding. I had thought that placing the baby on my chest would not be possible after a C-section. However, Jenny reassured me that it was possible.

At 37 weeks my baby was still breech, but there was still a hope it could turn. I visited one of the natural labour rooms and hoped that I would be able to deliver naturally in that room. We then toured the brightly lit and clinical theatre where C-sections were performed. As I had just seen the calm and soothing natural labour rooms, this was quite a shock. However, having seen it and been prepared for the operating theatre, I knew what to expect when the day of the C-section came and the delivery was a wonderfully positive experience for my husband and I. Somehow knowing what to expect and knowing exactly when my baby would arrive made us very calm. Everyone, from the obstetrician (Professor Bennett), to the anaesthetist (Felicity Plaat) and Jenny, was explaining what was happening at every step and I felt at ease.

When my baby was born I was asked if I knew the sex of my baby, which I did not, so they held him up for me to see. They then lay him on my chest. My wonderful baby snuggled into my neck, a feeling I will never forget. We were given the skin-to-skin time, which was so important to me. Within 30 minutes of his being born, Jenny helped me position my son to my breast and he fed greedily. I couldn't have asked for a more positive birth experience.'

BERNADETTE, 35

'Natural' Caesarean

The Natural Caesarean was an idea conceived by my colleague Professor Nicholas Fisk at Queen Charlotte's Hospital, and developed by both Felicity Plaat, a consultant anaesthetist and myself. The idea has been hugely popular with parents and, since its introduction, it has been taken up by hospitals across the country.

The central idea of the Natural Caesarean is to make the process less like an operation and to introduce some of the 'natural' aspects of a vaginal birth. This is achieved by allowing parents to be far more involved in the process. The actual operation, carried out by a surgeon, is exactly the same as a traditional Caesarean and there are no risks to the mother or baby.

In a traditional Caesarean section operation, there is a drape blocking the mother's view, so she cannot see her baby emerging from her uterus. With the Natural Caesarean, we do away with the screen and allow the mother to watch the baby being born. This means that the parents meet their baby at the same time as the operating team – with no missed moments. Mother and baby can bond through eye contact as the slow birth progresses. She can watch the birth of one arm, then the other, followed by the baby's body, gently supported by the surgeon. She can witness and cherish all these wonderful moments of birth and the baby is immediately placed skin to skin on her chest. The baby can then even begin breastfeeding while their mother is still on the operating table.

The Natural Caesarean is only suitable if your pregnancy is full term and your baby's head is down. It is not suitable for a breech or preterm baby, as the delay in the birthing process could put some babies at risk.

If you would like a Natural Caesarean, first discuss it with your obstetrician – it is definitely a procedure that needs a collaborative approach. Below I have listed the key points.

⊙ Tell your obstetrician, anaesthetist and midwife that you would like a Natural Caesarean.
⊙ Write it into your birth plan, including all the points you wish to discuss in advance.
⊙ Ask to see the operating theatre. If that isn't possible, ask to see a picture or video to give you an idea of what to expect from your surroundings.
⊙ Ask if the surgical team will play your own music and if your birth partner can take photographs.

On the day, you can expect the operation to be as described below.

⊙ The whole surgical team to be on board. This is essential. The procedure requires the collaboration of parents, surgeons, anaesthetist, midwife, scrub nurse, anaesthetic nurse and running nurse.
⊙ You will be given an epidural.
⊙ Once you hear the gurgling of the amniotic waters being released from the uterus, your theatre bed will be raised at the head and the screen/drape will be dropped so that you can witness your baby being born.
⊙ Your baby will be passed directly to you for immediate skin-to-skin contact.

The nurses will cover you in towels and bubble wrap to keep the baby warm (the air currents make operating theatres more drafty than labour rooms).

⊙ The father can then perform a second 'cutting of the cord' while the baby is in the mother's arms. The midwife will show him how to clamp the cord.

⊙ All the other procedures, such as labelling, carrying out head measurements and health and wellbeing checks can take place while the baby is enjoying skin-to-skin contact with the mother.

⊙ Checking the baby's weight will be delayed – it can be done when the mother is transferred from the operating table to her recovery bed.

If you decide for any reason that you want to change the procedure (for example, you want the drape raised and only dropped momentarily), do let your team know. It's still your choice, even once the surgery has begun.

If at any stage there are concerns about the welfare of the mother or the baby, the team will revert to traditional medical procedures.

CASE STUDY **NATURAL CAESAREAN**

'Mark and I were delighted when we were told that I was pregnant. Very early in my pregnancy I was told that, as a result of my age, I should be aware that I might need a Caesarean. As I was extremely squeamish, I wondered how women could cope with being conscious during such major surgery, and how I could persuade the hospital to give me my Caesarean under general anaesthetic.

I realized that I needed to work on my feelings and Mark and I, although initially sceptical, completed a Hypnobirthing and visualisation course. Both with this course and all the positive encouragement from my midwife Jenny, we started to see the day of the Caesarean as an amazing day where we would finally meet Noah, our baby, rather than the day of a serious operation. The Natural Caesarean was an extension of this positive approach, as the emphasis for us would be on both of us being together and watching Noah slowly emerge into the world for the first time.

Mark and I were shown the theatre where my Caesarean would take place.

When I first went in I felt relaxed and comfortable in the theatre. However, although my head was saying everything would be okay, I started to shake and I realized that I still needed to work on my feelings.

Jenny lent us a video of a Natural Caesarean, which showed us what to expect and reassured us that we would not see the incision or any blood. It was very important for me to discuss my fears and concerns with the obstetrician Professor Fisk and the anaesthetist beforehand and this helped to build up my confidence again. The anaesthetist kindly agreed to have a canister of gas and air in theatre for me, in the event of me having a wobble on the day of the Caesarean. They all agreed that, during the procedure, I could play a relaxing CD and I could take in geranium essence to mask the medical theatre smell.

On the day, the theatre staff made us feel we were participating in a beautiful family experience. Everyone was friendly and reassuring while the obstetrician made the incision. Once I heard the gurgling noises Jenny had described, I realized that the obstetrician had got through to my womb and that I could now see Noah being born. With Mark by my side, they lowered the screen and raised my head so that I could see Noah's little head poking out from my tummy. At first he gurgled to clear the fluid from his lungs, then he took his first breath followed by a healthy cry. Once he had fully emerged, Jenny handed him to me and he lay on me. The screen was then put up again. The immediate bonding was so exciting that I was virtually unaware of the surgery that followed. I did not use the gas and air but it was very reassuring to know that it was there and that the theatre staff were considering how I was going to feel throughout the procedure. I am sure that my quick recovery following the Caesarean was dramatically aided by the birth being such a positive experience.'

HARRIET, 44

types of obstetric pain relief

You may have decided that you want to use drugs during labour, or you may not be intending to use them. Whatever your choice, try to keep an open mind when it comes to pain relief in a first labour and, if necessary, factor a possible change of course into your birth plan.

There are many factors that can influence the level of pain you will feel:

⊙ the length of your labour
⊙ the size of your baby
⊙ whether you have an abnormal labour
⊙ how tired you are.

natural pain relief

There are many things you can do during labour to minimize the use of obstetric drugs, or do away with them completely. If you hope to avoid the use of painkilling drugs, see pages 236–40 for a list of natural methods for helping you through labour.

Labour without pain relief is perfectly possible for some women, particularly for those who have had a vaginal birth before. For others, the sheer power of the contractions can be overwhelming, making it very hard for them to maintain the idea of 'keeping your head stronger than your uterus' (see pages 71–3). In these cases, pain relief can get you back on track. Anyway, it is not a competition – if you need pain relief, you need pain relief. Once the pain relief is there, you can refocus and be mobile again. You can concentrate on the rest of labour and the journey to meet your baby. I think there are two things you need to take into account when you start thinking about pain relief:

⊙ where would I rate my pain threshold on a scale of 1 to 10?
⊙ where am I in my labour?

Pain relief comes in three forms:

⊙ inhaled drugs – gas and air (Entonox)
⊙ injections into your buttocks or leg – pethidine and diamorphine
⊙ injections into your back – epidural (spinal block).

gas and air (Entonox)

Entonox is the mildest of the three pain-relief options and can be a wonderful help in advanced labour and during the second stage. It's a combination of 50% oxygen and 50% nitrous oxide (laughing gas) and you are in control of the contraption that releases it, so you can introduce it as a ritual when you feel the contraction coming. It has fewer side effects than other obstetric painkillers and some women report it is more effective.

For some women, Entonox is amazingly helpful, particularly for those who have battled through most of the labour, are in the latter stages, and start to think 'I just can't go on now!' Entonox 'swims' them to the finishing line beautifully, in some cases.

The gas needs to be inhaled through the mouth by means of a mouthpiece or mask. In most hospitals, the supply is piped in the walls, but you can also receive it from cylinders, which usefully can be taken to home births.

For most effect, it is essential that the mother starts to breathe the gas in at the very beginning of the contraction so that the level of the gas reaches its peak just before the top of the contraction, where the pain is felt to be at its strongest. As the gas is breathed in, it goes into the lungs, then the bloodstream, and hits the thymus (the pain-controlling centre in the brain), reducing the sensation of pain at the top of the contraction. This leaves the mother with a warm sensation, often trickling up from the feet too, along with a slight woozy feeling in the head, which quickly resolves after gas is no longer breathed in after each contraction. It is very important that you breathe normal air between inhallations of Entonox to exhale the nitrous oxide.

Another point about Entonox is that it can provide a great distraction. While you are concentrating on breathing in at the right moment, you stop concentrating on the pain. The machine can then become part of a ritual to help you cope with contractions.

The advantage of the gas and air is that it can take the edge off the most intense part of the contraction and some women swear by it. The disadvantage is that it may not sustain you long term if you introduce it too early. Also, some women feel very nauseous (and even throw up) when they use it. It can also make your mouth and lips dry.

pethidine and diamorphine

These two separate drugs are both opoids (strong painkillers). Pethedine (meperide in the US) is widely available. Diamorphine is only used in the UK and South Africa. They are administered by injection into the thigh or bottom. They both take up to 45 minutes to work and last for 3–4 hours. As they cause nausea, you are usually given an anti-sickness injection at the same time. The best time to take pethidine is less than one hour before the birth, or more than four hours before.

Pethidine and diamorphine don't take away much pain at all, but alter your emotional response to pain, making you better able to cope with it. So you are still aware of the contractions and you can actively participate in the labour. However, both drugs, particularly pethidine, cross the placenta and can affect the baby – you won't be given either of these drugs if there is any chance you will give birth within one or two hours as they can cause breathing difficulties for the baby. Another disadvantage is that women often feel drowsy and disorientated and say they felt they 'lost' some of their labour as a result. Diamorphine can also make you itchy.

I rarely advocate these drugs for women in labour if other options (epidural) are available. I think they can make women lose the ability to 'make the head stronger than the uterus' (see pages 71–3) because they can end up feeling rather woozy, and are therefore not in control.

epidural

This is the most effective form of pain relief in labour and, if you are sure you want pain relief, this is the Rolls-Royce of obstetric drugs. It is also the most invasive and the most 'medicalized' (it is performed by an anaesthetist). You can't get away with just having the injection, you need an intravenous infusion, constant monitoring and, of course, it does have side effects.

In the UK, 22.5% of women receive an epidural in labour (this figure excludes the use in elective Caesareans), and they are usually used for first labours, induction (with syntocinon), mothers with high blood pressure and for Caesarean section. The rates vary from hospital to hospital, depending on the services provided, and in some places, it can be as high as 50% – even 70% in the private sector. The most common reason for an epidural to be given is on request, but in some cases it's recommended that you have one, for example if you have high blood pressure or you are expecting twins.

If you think that the pain you are experiencing is severe, and you are still a long way off the second stage, you may start to think about having an epidural.

Women who want to try a drug-free birth often ask for an epidural late in labour. A woman who is given an epidural at this late stage may not get any benefit from it, and the procedure itself can make her more panicky, as it is more difficult to insert the needle into a woman who is in pain and finding it difficult to curl up into and maintain the position required for insertion than it is to insert it into a woman who is not in as much pain. In my experience, nearly all women ask for an epidural at the point when they feel a pushing downwards. This is the exact stage when it is almost over. It might be that your partner or midwife needs to gently remind you, perhaps with energetic encouragement, positive support and love, that you are about to meet your wonderful baby. In many cases this is all that is needed to get you to push the baby out.

However – and this is a big however – no woman should be denied an epidural where it is possible, if this is what she wants. I have heard stories from mothers who felt the epidural they had asked for had been 'withheld'. One mother told me that she honestly believed her obstetrician had refused to give her this pain relief because he wanted to keep his epidural rate down on paper and keep his 'natural birth' credentials intact. While this may have been a confusion of communication, the fact is that she was traumatized by the experience. Another mother came to me for her second birth saying her first had been terrible. When she recounted the details, I said 'but that sounds like a wonderful experience.' She shook her head vigorously, 'I wasn't allowed an epidural.' She asked me to write in her medical notes that she must have an epidural as soon as possible. I agreed. This mother felt strongly that the 'head stronger than the uterus' ideal wasn't for her. Perhaps she felt her head didn't work like that. But it was her choice. When she went into labour with her second baby, we gave her the epidural she wanted, exactly when she wanted it. She had all the magic moments with her baby. Afterwards she described it as her 'perfect birth'. she said she would even consider having more children – something that had previously been unthinkable.

So the decision is yours.

THE PROCEDURE

First you are given an intravenous infusion. This is because the epidural can lower your blood pressure and cause you to feel faint and reduce blood flow to the baby. Then the anaesthetist will administer the epidural. Positioning is key here. The anaesthetist will usually ask you to sit cross-legged on the edge of the bed, relax your shoulders and arch your back 'like an angry cat', so that the vertebrae in your back open up. It is important to stay in a level position – don't tilt to one side. Obviously, this is easier said than done – your abdomen is full of baby and you may also be getting very regular contractions. Many units suggest a foetal position with the mother lying on her left side.

Your back will then be sprayed with antiseptic spray, which is freezing cold. The doctor, who will now be masked and gowned, will have a sterile trolley. He or she will feel your back to find best the place to insert the epidural (or spinal block). He or she will apply a local anaesthetic to your skin in order to numb it, then you will feel a pushing feeling, which is the needle going into your back. You will feel a fair amount of pressure in your back, so you must be still. It's best to let the doctor know if you are getting contractions so that the needle does not go in too far. If available, you can use the Entonox at this point to help you through the contractions.

Women are usually very surprised when they see the size of an epidural needle when they are not in labour, but for many it is a welcome sight in labour if they are finding it hard to cope with the pain. The epidural space is approximately 5–6cm below the skin. The needle is inserted between the backbones and 4cm of catheter is left in the epidural space itself. Once in, the anaesthetist will thread a thin plastic tube through the needle, then remove the needle. Dressings are put in place to ensure the tube is securely stuck in your back. You will then be attached to a CTG monitor for at least 30 minutes.

As the epidural begins to work you will feel a warm sensation going to your bottom. A good test if it is working well is if the mother doesn't feel any pain and both feet are warm if felt by the anaethetist or midwife. If one foot is cooler it can mean the little catheter has moved a little to the side. You may need to lie of the side of the cooler foot to even it out.

Further 'top-ups' are given through this tube usually one to two hourly (usually by the midwife) but sometimes every 30 minutes. While you will often receive continuous monitoring by CTG, you can just ask for 30 minutes straight after the 'top up'. You will have your blood pressure checked regularly and it may drop during the procedure – which can make you faint and reduce the blood flow to the baby. Although rare in labour, this is one reason for keeping up the fluid in your blood stream via an intravenous infusion.

DISADVANTAGES

One of the main disadvantages of the epidural during labour is that it can make it difficult for you to push the baby out because you can't feel your perineum. I recommend that you try to get some of the pressure feeling back – although not the pain (as it is counter productive) – so that you can focus on where to bear down in the pushing stage. You can use upright positions to do this, or a birth stool, which is great until your baby's head is visible. It also greatly reduces the chance of a ventouse or forceps delivery (see pages 269–72). Most epidurals in labour will be of a type that allows maximum mobility. The drug used contains very little marcain, which causes numbness, and a larger dose of fentanyl, a painkiller; with so little marcain, women can still walk around. In cases of C-section and sometimes forceps or ventouse, a higher dose of marcain is given, making women unable to move for a while, or pass urine.

Other disadvantages are the possible side effects:

- ⊙ 4% of women experience incomplete pain relief, for example you may feel anaesthetized down one side but still have pain in the other
- ⊙ itching
- ⊙ nausea and vomiting
- ⊙ backache after the birth (in some cases this can be severe)
- ⊙ bladder dysfunction after birth – it's for this reason that I emphasize the importance of going to the loo before each top up. An epidural can make it difficult for you to pass urine and this can cause distension of the bladder
- ⊙ there is an increased chance of instrumental vaginal delivery.

Horror stories about permanent paralysis abound, but this is actually extremely rare, as are allergic shock and convulsions. A urinary catheter to help you empty the bladder may be advised.

COMBINED EPIDURAL/SPINAL

This is a combination of the epidural and spinal block, as they work together quickly. It is also known as the mobile epidural. The advantages of being mobile are that it may help to progress labour and you may be more comfortable moving around or adopting an upright position for birth.

THE SPINAL ANAESTHETIC

This is used for speed when a full block is needed and an epidural is not already in situ. The procedure is similar to that of the epidural, but the injection is put in at a slightly different location. It is used for Caesarian sections, forceps deliveries, ventouse deliveries or alongside epidurals, where it works most effectively.

INCREASING YOUR CHANCES OF A VAGINAL BIRTH

The best way to maximize your chance of delivering your baby vaginally if you have an epidural, and without the aid of forceps or ventouse, is to follow this advice. Have a top-up at the beginning of the second stage and wait for the feeling of pressure that you'll feel in your bottom. If you have had a mobile epidural, walk around, sit on a rocking chair or use a birth stool to encourage the baby's head to descend. When you feel strong pressure, push during each contraction, which will cause an increased sensation in the vagina/bottom.

When your baby's head can be seen constantly, get onto all fours on a mat. This will reduce the pressure on the perineum and control the delivery of the head and shoulders, reducing the chances of tearing or needing an episiotomy.

Of course, if your baby's heart rate is abnormal, you will need to deliver quickly, in which case forceps or ventouse may be needed.

If you have to lie on a bed, try to keep moving your body, wriggling if necessary, to avoid getting sore patches of skin caused by lying in one position for too long.

second time around

If this is not your first baby, it is worth knowing that second and subsequent births can be very different experiences. For example, many women think that, because their first one was early or late, the second one will be too. This is not always the case.

Second babies are, statistically, the safest and easiest in terms of labour and delivery, and the chance of having a Caesarean section after a natural first birth is greatly reduced. However, if you have an undiagnosed breech or a placenta abruption (when the placenta separates from the wall of the uterus), you will be rushed to theatre. Third babies are often described as 'unpredictable'; fourth ones as 'fast' and fifth as 'early' – but, of course, there is no definite rule with birth.

the risk factor of previous complications

If you encountered complications during a previous pregnancy, then at the beginning of your current pregnancy you need to discuss your risks with your doctor or midwife. Below is a list of common first-time complications and the associated risk in a second pregnancy.

- ⊙ Pre-eclampsia
  40% chance. The risk of having it again is actually around 20%, but specialists cite a range of 5–80%, depending on a number of factors including severity in the first instance and number of times you have been affected.
- ⊙ Premature birth
  15% chance of having another baby early, or to put it more positively, 85% chance of having your next baby at term (or even overdue).
- ⊙ Gestational diabetes
  45% chance.
- ⊙ Pregnancy-induced hypertension
  Now called gestational or transient hypertension or chronic hypertension. 50% chance. (This is caused by high blood pressure and the problem

occurs in late pregnancy without any of the signs of pre-eclampsia. It can indicate blood pressure problems later in life.)

- ⊙ Baby that is small for dates
  8% chance.
- ⊙ 'Assisted' delivery
  For example, ventouse, forceps etc – about a 22% chance.
- ⊙ Caesarean first time
  24–28% chance if you are trying for a vaginal birth second time around (see the notes on VBAC below).

vaginal birth after Caesarean (VBAC)

Obviously your chances of success at having a VBAC depend to a great extent on what happened in your first labour. If your cervix didn't open first time around, your birth will be more similar to that of a first time mother. If you managed to dilate to 5cm before hitting a problem in the first labour, you have a better chance than if your cervix didn't open last time. If you reached second stage (the pushing stage) first time around, you have around an 80% chance of a successful vaginal birth.

If you had a Caesarean because, for example, your baby was breech, it may be the shape of your pelvis that is an issue. It is more common, however, for a first baby to be occipito posterior (see page 103), and many women have no problem progressing second time around.

My feeling with women who have failed to progress is that, second time around, the baby has got more chance of turning into a favourable position because the abdominal muscles are more distended and softer, allowing the baby to turn more comfortably.

THE BENEFITS OF A VAGINAL BIRTH

- ⊙ You avoid the risks associated with surgery.
- ⊙ You will have a quicker and less painful recovery than with a Caesarean.
- ⊙ You don't need to be in the hospital for as long.
- ⊙ It reduces the incidence of breathing difficulties for the baby – as the baby goes through labour its lungs are prepared for birth.
- ⊙ It is safer in the long run if you want more than two children.

The more Caesareans you have, the higher the risk to you and to the baby. The scar is more likely to rupture, the placenta is more likely to stick to the scar and it's more likely for the placenta to be at the front. There is also an accompanying risk of stillbirth if you have more than three Caesarean sections. If, however, you have had a vaginal birth, then a C-section, then a VBAC, you have a 90% chance of a normal birth fourth time around.

THE RISKS OF VBAC

- ☉ Overall, you have an approximately 70% chance of having a normal vaginal birth but a 30% chance of having an emergency C-section (which carries higher risks than a planned Caesarean section). This can be hugely disappointing and distressing, especially if it is a long labour.
- ☉ You may be more at risk if there was a shorter delivery time between your last baby and this pregnancy (less than two years).
- ☉ The scar ruptures in approximately 1 in 200 deliveries.
- ☉ 3 in 1,000 chance of a huge scar rupture which results in a hysterectomy – (the risk of a mother who has had one past Caesarean section ending up with a hysterectomy is 1 in 90).
- ☉ The risk of foetal death is 1 in 3,500.

SCAR RUPTURE We usually suspect a scar is about to rupture when women start complaining of 'pain all the time'. If the scar does then rupture, the mother may get referred shoulder pain because the blood that comes out of the scar irritates the diaphragm.

If you are determined to have a VBAC, there are a few things to remember from the outset. Tell your obstetrician as soon as possible and discuss with them what happened in your previous pregnancy. Give as detailed a history as possible of your last labour. It's important that you are considered as an individual case because your last experience will have a bearing on what to expect second time around. Avoid having a Caesarean scheduled at 39 weeks as a backup (most women have not gone into labour by then so you are more likely to end up with another Caesarean).

In most cases, VBAC is a birth choice. Your obstetrician will give you the information you need. My advice is that you must make your decision while completely understanding all the inherent risks for your individual case.

In some cases your obstetrician will strongly advise against it, even if you are adamant. This may happen if you:

- had a vertical Caesarean the first time (i.e. an 'up and down' scar as opposed to a bikini scar)
- had a T-incision (in which the uterus is cut both horizontally and vertically)
- have already had two previous Caesareans
- had previously attempted a VBAC and your scar had ruptured. In this case you would not be allowed to try again.

the run-up to labour

The run-up to labour can feel like waiting for a night bus. You know it's going to arrive, but when? Be reassured – you won't miss it! Go with the flow; think happy thoughts of meeting your gorgeous baby and allow the final phase of your pregnancy run its course.

practical preparations

Pregnant women waiting for the birth of their first child often feel as if time is standing still – even going backwards – in the last month of pregnancy. Giving yourself things to do that are directly linked to your labour will be a welcome distraction – and very useful. Your partner may be able to take on preparations for labour and your baby's arrival, which can help him feel more involved.

planning your trip to the hospital

You don't need nice smart things in labour, but you may want a couple of 'luxuries' that are personal to you. In my case, during all my labours I held on to my pashmina shawl and had a wet flannel on my face to close everyone else out. I have met a woman who brought an amaryllis flower onto the labour ward for her first labour, and a cabbage for the second. I've also seen women take their husband's pyjama tops or wash their labour clothes in advance so that they have the familiar smell of home.

ADDITIONAL ESSENTIALS
In addition to your hospital bag (see page 225), there are a few essentials you need to remember. Some women put a checklist by the front door to make sure they have everything, but basically these are:

- ⊙ the baby's car seat (you may want to fit this in advance)
- ⊙ your obstetric (hospital) notes
- ⊙ your birth plan
- ⊙ change for the car park
- ⊙ plastic sheet for the back seat
- ⊙ sign for the dashboard to say you have been rushed into the labour ward
- ⊙ change for the telephone.

WHAT DO I NEED TO ORGANIZE?
Forward planning for labour is a good idea – you don't know when it's going to happen, you don't know how long you may be kept in for. Think about and plan

for the following issues in advance.

- ⊙ Who will take care of your other children? This needs to be someone who can be 'on call' 24 hours and who lives relatively close to your house. Someone may need to take your children to school in the morning, too.
- ⊙ Who is caring for your pets?
- ⊙ Does a neighbour have a key in case of emergencies?

WHAT MODE OF TRANSPORT SHOULD I TAKE?

TAXI If you're taking a taxi, make sure that the company you use takes women who are in labour (some won't), you have the number close at hand, you take a spare towel and that you have some plastic for the car seat (much like the mattress protector, this will limit damage if, say, your waters break en route; even a bin bag will offer some protection).

CAR If you're going in the car, it's a good idea to make sure that the person taking you knows the route, that they are not over the legal drink-drive limit, you have some plastic for the car seat to protect from possible damage (if your waters break) and that you know how to get to the hospital car park (if there is one). Money for the car park will be useful. Also make sure you know how to get to the labour ward, you know the 'out of hours' procedures (many labours happen at night) and you have an emergency note for the dashboard to let parking wardens know you have been rushed to the labour ward. Sometimes there just isn't time to park. Don't bring up your bag and equipment straightaway if you are in a rush – your partner can return for the luggage once they have deposited you in the hands of midwives on the labour ward.

PUBLIC TRANSPORT If you are banking on public transport, you'll need to think a few things through. While you may have time in a first labour to take a bus or train to the hospital, public transport can be hit by sudden problems. You don't want labour to advance rapidly while you wait for a broken-down bus to be repaired, for example. Public transport can be unreliable in the middle of the night, at weekends or on public holidays. You will probably need to organize an emergency back-up plan, whether it be a lift from a friend, family member or a taxi. Only use an ambulance in an emergency – they are not a taxi service.

WHAT DO I NEED TO KNOW ON THE LABOUR WARD?

Once you are safely delivered to the hospital, you'll need to get your bearings. Perhaps this is something for your partner to think about. He can ask your care providers in advance the following questions: who is my allocated midwife? Where will she be in an emergency? Where is the nearest staff station to my room? Where is the emergency bell (in most cases you won't need it, but it's better to know where it is just in case)? Where is the loo? Where can I get water? Where can I get tea and coffee? Where can I leave the car on a long-term basis?

your hospital bag

What you take with you to the hospital is a personal choice, but there are some basics everyone should have, such as:

For you:
- ⊙ nightie or a T-shirt
- ⊙ eye mask – invaluable for blocking out unwanted bright lights
- ⊙ face cloths/ flannels
- ⊙ lip salve – provides great relief from dry lips if you have gas and air
- ⊙ tennis balls, which are very useful if you have a 'back labour', because your partner can rub the base of the spine with the ball
- ⊙ lavender oil, or any other oils you like
- ⊙ a scarf – you may become cold in labour; you can also use it to wrap yourself up in and shut out the world
- ⊙ your own pillow (so much nicer than the ones at the hospital)
- ⊙ 'snuggly bits' – personal items that make you feel comfortable and comforted, such as a photo of your

children, a picture to help with your visualisations, your husband's shirt
- ⊙ socks (feet can get suddenly cold)
- ⊙ old fashioned sanitary towels
- ⊙ water spray
- ⊙ water bottles or little cartons of juice
- ⊙ snacks (in a low-risk labour that is progressing normally, you need to eat little and often); nuts and dried fruit are good choices, as are high-energy snack bars (taste them first – not all are nice) and glucose tablets
- ⊙ CD player and music or Hypnobirthing CDs
- ⊙ camera
- ⊙ this book.

For your baby:
- ⊙ newborn-size nappies
- ⊙ sleep suits (babygros)
- ⊙ vests
- ⊙ hat
- ⊙ cardigan, socks, mittens (if it's cold)
- ⊙ scratch mitts.

signs that labour is approaching

'WARM-UP' CONTRACTIONS (OR 'FALSE LABOUR')

Braxton Hicks contractions (see pages 91 and 138–9) move up a gear as labour approaches, and you may start to find them uncomfortable. In some women they start to cause a tightening sensation in the bottom, too, in some, their lower backs and, occasionally, some women feel them at the top of the uterus first.

You may find you get 'runs' of Braxton Hicks in the evening or even at night, where you experience contractions coming every five minutes for half an hour before they tail off again. You may think that this is the start of labour. One way to tell is to get up – 'false contractions' will usually subside if you walk around.

I often get calls from women wondering if they are in labour – and I sometimes wash my hair in preparation for a long night of work, only to find I am still in bed in the morning.

when the baby's head is 'engaged'

If your midwife or doctor tells you that your baby's head is engaged, it means that the widest part of the head has descended into your pelvis. They can tell this by feeling your baby's head through the abdomen. I try to explain it to women in my care by getting them to imagine the baby's head in five sections. If I can no longer feel the first three sections of the baby's head in the abdomen, then that baby is 'engaged'.

Basically, this means that preparation for birth is in its final stages. When the baby's head is engaged, it will stay there. You will often hear the moment of engagement referred to as 'lightening' and some women say they can even feel the moment of lightening. It is more profound in first pregnancies because you can visibly see where your uterus has dropped from being high above your rib cage to almost a shelf you can balance a cup of tea on!

The momentary relief you will feel in your rib cage may, however, be replaced by discomfort lower down as the baby's head comes to rest on your bladder.

This is when you start needing to go to the loo more often and you may get tweaks and twinges in your vagina.

If you are feeling heaviness or swelling in the pelvic area – particularly towards the end of the day – this is most likely to be caused by the increased fluid gathering in your soft tissues, and is due to the baby's weight and gravity. For relief, get your legs and feet in a position where they are above your pelvis.

If a first baby's head has not engaged, the midwife will try to find out why. It could be something as simple as a full bladder – this can make a baby's head stay 'up'. Other reasons for a baby's head not to engage include the presence of a low-lying placenta, an ovarian cyst or a fibroid. Most of these concerns will have been pre-diagnosed by those looking after you.

Second and subsequent babies may not engage until the onset of labour and, generally speaking, that is not a cause for concern. They may start labour with their heads still relatively high in the abdomen but, as contractions get stronger, the head usually drops quickly.

I add one warning: if your baby's head hasn't engaged and your waters break with a big gush prior to labour, you need to call an ambulance. You are not in danger of the baby arriving unless contractions start. If they do, get yourself into what is called the 'knee-chest' position (see page 242).

The main reason for this position is as a precaution against a cord prolapse (when the umbilical cord drops before the baby's head), which is very rare and occurs only when the cervix has already opened and there is space for the cord to drop.

There is usually enough time to get to hospital before your cervix has opened and you are at any risk of a cord prolapse. If you are worried, however, call the labour ward and seek help from the midwives.

◁ The baby's head is engaged when the top of the head descends into the pelvic cavity, ready for delivery.

being overdue

Before you worry about going overdue, you should remember that the vast majority of women go over their due date with their first pregnancy. On average, first time babies are born five days past the due date, with 10% going beyond 42 weeks (compared to 4% born on their due date).

The current process for calculating due dates was devised at the beginning of the 19th century by Dr Franz Naegele, a German obstetrician. Naegele's Rule estimates the due date from the last missed period (LMP), adding a year, subtracting three months and adding seven days (another way of working it out is by adding 266 days to the date of conception – i.e. day 14). However, this idea is based on the premise that a menstrual cycle is 28 days and ovulation occurs on day 14. It does not take into account that some women have longer or shorter cycles, nor does it take into account diet, age or previous pregnancies.

Indeed, there are many factors that will influence your actual gestation period, not least your ethnic origin. Some studies suggest we should add a further two weeks to that date for first-time Caucasian mothers, 10 days for Caucasian mothers on their second or subsequent pregnancies. One study suggests that African and Asian women tend to have shorter gestations – with a median gestational age at delivery of 39 weeks. Black women with a normal body mass index (BMI) were also found to have increased odds of preterm delivery.[17]

'natural' induction

There is a whole range of 'natural' methods to bring on labour. Most of these are worth a try because, if you end up being induced, at least you will know that you tried everything else beforehand. The majority of the following can be attempted anytime after 39 weeks:

- ⊙ acupuncture
- ⊙ reflexology
- ⊙ visualisation
- ⊙ sex, sex, sex and more sex (although this may be the last thing you feel

like, it can be effective)
- ⊙ eating curry
- ⊙ a glass of champagne
- ⊙ a long walk (although don't exhaust or over-exert yourself or you won't be able to cope with labour)
- ⊙ eating pineapple (these contain bromelain which is said to stimulate prostaglandin which helps make the cervix soften)
- ⊙ nipple stimulation (which can help release oxytocin, which is thought to help trigger labour).

cervical stretch

You can also ask your midwife to give you a 'cervical stretch' (also called a membrane sweep). This will often get labour going in a mother whose cervix has already begun to efface and dilate, and is approved by The Royal College of Obstetricians and Gynaecologists as a last option before the artificial induction of labour.

The procedure basically involves either the obstetrician or midwife stretching your cervix with their finger and trying to separate the membranes from the top of the cervix and lower uterine wall. If effective, labour will start within 48 hours.

It can feel a little uncomfortable, particularly if your cervix is set back. If simple relaxation techniques don't take away the discomfort you can ask for gas and air.

the big day

Your womb starts its own 'marathon', squeezing your baby down and down with each contraction. Take the contractions one by one. As each one ends, think to yourself that that's another one gone, and that you are another contraction closer to meeting your baby.

the onset of labour

Many women, first-time mothers in particular, are anxious that they won't be able to recognize when they are in labour. Experiencing one of the following symptoms is likely to be a sign that your big day is soon to, or has, arrived. You may experience more than one of these.

PERIOD-LIKE CRAMP

Some women have described having period-like cramps in the days (and, in a subsequent pregnancy, even weeks) before labour. This is an indication that your cervix is opening and effacing in preparation for labour. The cramps may start to go hand-in-hand with stronger runs of Braxton Hicks (see pages 91 and 138–9) and this can be an indication that labour is only days away.

A 'BLOODY SHOW'

You may experience a 'bloody show', which is the loss of your mucous plug, which closes off the cervix during pregnancy, creating a natural barrier betwen the uterus and the vagina. A show comes in many forms: it can be pinky, streaked with blood (blood vessels from the cervix can bleed as it opens), thick clear or opaque mucus, or thick gungy mucus that is discoloured, even brown.

signs that labour is approaching

Common signs are:
- period-like cramps
- a 'bloody show'
- sudden sensitivity to light and noise
- a desire to 'hide' or to be alone
- the baby's position changes/movements increase or decrease
- a sudden loss of appetite
- flu-like symptoms, diarrhoea, vomiting, a temperature
- waters breaking
- backache
- strong contractions.

A show is usually a sign that labour is not far away. It can still be days rather than hours, and for some women up to 10 days, so conserve your energy and try not to get too excited. You can also start labour without a show.

It should not be fresh red blood and it should not be dripping out like a period – if you experience anything like this you need to call your doctor or midwife as this can be indicative of placenta abruption (when the placenta comes away from the womb lining), which is an emergency situation.

A SUDDEN SENSITIVITY TO LIGHT AND NOISE

Again, not every woman experiences this, but this can be an instinctive, almost primal response to the onset of labour. As I've said throughout the book, many women like to dim the lights, they like the room to feel 'closed down' and they may suddenly feel averse to the noise of the television or people talking. If you have guests, you may suddenly want them to leave. If this is the case, it goes without saying that you should make your excuses and retreat to a place where you feel comfortable.

If you feel this very strongly as labour commences, you can use any number of props to help you shut out the outside world. I used a warm wet cloth, which I draped over my face to keep things dark. Some women prefer an eye mask, others a scarf.

A DESIRE TO 'HIDE' OR TO BE ALONE

This often goes hand-in-hand with the point above, in which case retreat to your 'sanctuary' (see pages 168–9), explaining to others your need to disappear. It can also begin to happen when labour is already in full swing.

As I have said before, some women start to heavily guard their privacy and have a need to feel safe; they may go behind a door during a contraction or retreat into a small dark room on their own, such as the loo or the shower, or even hide behind furniture.

Yehudi Gordon, in his book *Birth and Beyond*, stresses that women need to feel safe in order for oxytocin to flow, which in turn makes labour go more smoothly. I called it being 'snuggled'. Michel Odent points out that if you don't feel secure, adrenaline takes over and labour slows right down. For example, some women find their labours stop if they don't feel relaxed. It might be the presence of their partner or even an attendant they don't like in the room. Their labour may speed up once that person leaves or they retreat to another room.

This can occasionally be a problem for midwives. I've heard stories of women disappearing into the loo during the second stage and midwives knocking on the door trying to gently coax them out, while being fearful that the baby might actually be arriving.

A SUDDEN LOSS OF APPETITE

Some women suddenly experience weight loss of around 500g to a kilo in the week before labour begins. Although your appetite may have subsided significantly in the last couple of weeks (there is very little room left for your stomach), a sudden loss of appetite can signal that things are about to get going. One reason for this may be that your body is 'flushing out' in advance of labour. It could also be caused by the hormonal changes that take place before labour.

It is also a common reaction to contractions starting. Even if you feel like you can't face anything, try to eat little and often in labour – it can be a long journey and you need to keep your energy reserves high. I recommend nuts, energy bars, rice or oatcakes and even the glucose tablets (such as Dextrasol) used by athletes. If you really can't eat, you must at least try to drink – I recommend sports drinks with electrolytes.

It's important not to get very dehydrated as this can cause your baby's heart rate to increase.

FLU-LIKE SYMPTOMS, DIARRHOEA AND VOMITING

Diarrhoea is always a bit of a surprise for pregnant women, who spend so much time worrying about being constipated. As I said above, this is a sign that your body is 'flushing out', so that you begin labour with empty bowels. Similarly vomiting and a slightly raised temperature can be your body's way of ensuring the gastrointestinal tract is clear before labour starts. It can also be linked to hormonal changes. (If you have strong flu-like symptoms accompanied by a fever BEFORE the onset of labour, be sure to tell your doctor or midwife – you may actually have the flu!)

Some women also feel nauseous and pass wind and, in severe cases, have continued vomiting and diarrhoea throughout labour. This can also be caused by a reaction to Entonox (gas and air). You may also vomit later in labour, at 'transition' (see pages 256–7), and experience a rush of flu-like hot-and-cold shivers (which you can alleviate by either taking off clothes or putting on socks and a scarf). In this situation women often don't know if they want to throw up or open their bowels, but the feeling is usually short lived.

If you feel constant nausea in labour my advice is to have an injection to relieve it. Women have told me that the vomiting or constant nausea can be worse than contractions.

If you experience a temperature you should also have some form of pain relief (such as paracetamol) to bring it down. Epidurals can cause a spike in temperature in some women, but this often settles with an increase in the intravenous fluid, which is set up before you have the injection.

WATERS BREAKING

It always happens in the films, but it is far less common in real life. Only 10–15% of women experience their waters breaking in advance of labour. It can be a dramatic event when your waters break, with amniotic fluid literally gushing forth – the 'flooded swimming pool' effect. You may also experience just a small trickle of fluid and be unsure whether that really was your waters breaking. This is usually because the baby's head is acting like a cork in a bottle and preventing a more dramatic amount of fluid loss. (If you are unsure whether or not your waters have gone, go to the loo, dry yourself and then wear a sanitary towel. If, after a few mintues, it is wet, then it is most likely that your waters have broken.) Amniotic fluid smells very different to urine (it has a sweet odour) and it is colourless.

If your waters do break, you may suddenly experience contractions. Other women experience a delay before their contractions start and, in some cases, have to be induced. You need to contact your doctor or midwife if your waters break as you are slightly at risk from infection. Don't go swimming if your waters have broken.

Most women only see their waters go towards the second stage when the baby's head pressing down puts pressure on the amniotic sac. At the end of pregnancy you can have as little as two tea cups of amniotic fluid left around the baby – or as much as six, but in some labours you barely see any waters. In very rare cases babies can be born with their amniotic sac intact – this is called a 'caul' (see page 259).

If you are worried about your waters breaking at an untimely moment, keep a spare pair of knickers and a few sanitary pads in your handbag, so you can't be caught off guard.

BACKACHE

This symptom has made an appearance at every stage in pregnancy and, once again, it can return to be a symptom of the onset of labour. It may be even more noticeable if you haven't experienced any backache up until now. The backache may be constant, with regular bouts of stronger back pain. I discuss how to treat backache in labour with natural remedies (see pages 237 and 240). Use these guidelines to help you through the early stages of labour.

what is a contraction?

The uterus is made up of interlaced muscle fibres. When the muscle fibres at the top shorten, your uterus contracts (often sending pain and pressure into your lower back and front). When the muscles relax, the fibres remain short, keeping pressure at the top of the uterus, but allowing the bottom of the uterus (the neck of the womb) to become thinner and to dilate.

The repetition of this action pushes your baby downwards and causes the cervix to open further, rather like as if you were to force the baby's head through a too-tight polo-neck jumper. The continued pressure on your cervix opens the neck of the uterus and the baby is able to descend through the boney passageways of the birth canal, until he or she reaches the soft tissues of the pelvic floor.

STRONG CONTRACTIONS

I heard someone describe a contraction as having the strings of a corset pulled very suddenly and very hard and, in some cases, it feels exactly like that. However, women 'feel' contractions differently.

In my experience, first labours start quite slowly and gently. The uterus has a few bursts of activity, then settles down. This can go on for some time (and be quite frustrating) until there are regular strong contractions, coming for two to three minutes every 10 minutes or more, that literally take your breath away.

The general rule of midwives and obstetricians alike is that if a woman cannot speak during a contraction, they are in 'true' labour. If they are having regular contractions every three minutes, 'established' labour has arrived.

Not all women find labour painful – some describe it as 'mildly painful', some as 'intense'. Everyone is different and may be influenced by different factors – from past experience of pain, to feelings of fear or tension.

managing pain in early labour

Even if you plan to have an epidural at some point, arming yourself with tools for the onset of labour and the early hours will help you stay calm, together and in control. You will also be able to labour at home for longer, which reduces the risk of being sent home from the hospital if your labour isn't far enough advanced. Once you have got into the swing of some of the ideas below, you will probably find your labour is progressing manageably and you may decide you don't need any other form of pain relief.

natural pain relief

Below I have adapted a list of tools for 'natural pain relief'. These are from Penny Simkin, a well-respected American writer on childbirth (see page 329). I have added my own notes and the wisdom of others in the field of childbirth to give you the broadest possible advice.

THE BATH

The combined effects of warmth and skin stimulation from water are soothing and relaxing. Simkin cites studies that show how getting into a bath when you are in 'active labour' (approximately 3cm dilated) significantly helps relieve pain and lowers blood pressure, but warns that you should keep the water just above body temperature. If you are planning to give birth in the water, it is recommended that you use the birthing pool when your labour is more advanced (you are 5cm+ dilated).

SHOWER

The benefits of a shower include warmth, privacy and the fact that it has a lovely hypnotic sound. Training a shower onto your lower back can also be hugely comforting if you have a strong 'back' labour.

TENS MACHINE

TENS is short for transcutaneous electrical nerve stimulation. This is a hand-held device that is powered by battery, which means you can use it at home from early in labour and still move around (although you can't use it in the bath or shower).

It works by transmitting electrical impulses through your skin via pads that stick onto your back. As labour pain increases, so you can increase the intensity of the impulses. For this reason you need to start it early on. It can also act as a distraction and become a 'ritual' as, each time you feel the contraction coming on you can press the booster button.

The electrodes interrupt pain messages to your brain and, according to some, increase the production of natural endorphins. Studies show that it reduces and postpones the use of epidurals and some women find it highly beneficial.

It's best to hire a TENS machine rather than buy one. Hire it in advance, at about 37 weeks. (See page 329 for details of where to hire one.)

PRESSURE APPLIED BY YOUR PARTNER

Simkin suggests three types of pressure for labour pain in the sacroiliac joints (lower back):

⊙ your partner applies pressure on your lower back throughout each contraction (this can also be done with a tennis ball or rolling pin) with one hand, and holds you around the front of the pelvis to help steady you, with the other
⊙ your partner pushes the top of your buttocks together throughout each contraction
⊙ if you sit down with your back straight and your feet elevated on a cushion, your partner, kneeling in front of you, cups your knees and presses them back towards your hips.

HOT AND COLD PACKS

Hot water bottles are a well-known remedy for helping back, shoulder and lower-abdomen pain in labour, but they can be doubled up with cold packs for greater effect. The heat increases circulation and reduces tension; the cold numbs and relieves muscle spasm, which in turn provides pain relief.

MASSAGE AND TOUCH

Repetition is a natural human way of coping with stressful or intense situations – something I call 'the rituals of labour' (see page 240). In the same way, rhythmical stroking of the shoulders, back, arms and legs can be very soothing and comforting in labour.

Obstetrician Michel Odent believes that natural endorphins flow stronger when a woman is feeling secure and loved, and even simple gestures, such as hand holding, a light foot massage or being held close, can be hugely beneficial in this way.

I should add here that some women do not like to be touched or approached in labour as they find it distracting.

ACUPUNCTURE, REFLEXOLOGY AND ACUPRESSURE

Acupuncture and reflexology can be used for natural induction of labour. They can also be an effective pain relief. Some doulas are also qualified in these areas so can practise these ancient arts while you are in labour.

SELF-COMFORTING TECHNIQUES

As Simkin says, 'these techniques are some of the mainstays of the self-comforting measures for labour'. They are also the corner stone of most antenatal and pregnancy yoga classes in the UK and, in some cases, what women find they do naturally in labour – when they feel calm, secure and in control. I can't emphasize enough how important it is to practise self-comforting techniques in advance of labour, so they are almost second nature to you when the day arrives.

FOCUSING Women often focus on an object or spot on the wall when they are seized by the intensity of a contraction. Here I like to introduce my Swirls (see page 169) as something women can focus on and use as an illustration of the contraction as well as a way of coping with it.

BREATHING In pregnancy yoga, Pilates and Hypnobirthing, women are taught the importance of concentrating on slow, regular breathing. See page 74 for suggestions of how you can practise pattern breathing.

RELAXATION TECHNIQUES Simple techniques such as consciously 'softening your jaw' and concentrating on 'widening the gap between your shoulders and your ears' are, in themselves, hugely helpful in the face of an intense contraction. Keep in mind Dick-Read's discussion on the relationship between fear, tension and pain (see page 68). If you can eliminate the fear and tension, you will go a long way to easing the pain.

VISUALISATION I have discussed visualisation on pages 71–73, 128 and 168. This is one of the most effective tools of all for getting through labour. Almost all childbirth specialists advocate visualisations for labour and they are most effective if thought about and practised in advance. The Hypnobirthing movement suggests visualising the act of 'releasing' or 'letting go', and you can incorporate this to help you relax even more completely.

SELF-HYPNOSIS This has become extremely popular in recent years and I have seen the results – it is highly effective. The Hypnobirthing movement, which is an American organization that now operates in the UK (see page 329 for their website address), teaches self-hypnosis through a combination of breathing, visualisation and 'birthing affirmations' – positive thoughts that you practise in advance and then repeat during labour.

HYPNOSIS/ BIRTHING CDS These are now available from a number of different sources, including my colleague Gowri Motha. Some teach self-hypnosis for birth. The CDs usually combine hypnosis and music and lull you into a wonderfully calm state. See page 329 for sources.

EMOTIONAL PROPS OR 'SNUGGLY BITS' These are familiar items that you can bring with you in labour to make the hospital or birth-centre environment more personal. These can be any number of things – a photograph of your family or a place you love, a favourite pillow, a soft shawl, oils, your husband's shirt, a favourite teddy, a stress ball, a lavender bag, even illustrations of a baby moving down the birth canal.

MUSIC For those that find music relaxing, it can be a huge comfort during labour, especially a familiar piece of music that has seen them through their pregnancy.

VOCALIZING Women make quite primal noises as their labour carries them into the second stage. It's important to keep these noises deep, almost like cattle lowing, and not high, which could put you at risk of hyperventilating. If you prastise pregnancy yoga, you might have been taught to sound the 'Om', which resonates in the pelvis, abdomen, chest and throat. This might be a useful sound for vocalizing effectively during labour.

RITUALS 'The rituals' are what I call the repetitive actions of women in labour. Once women have found something that has comforted them through a contraction (be it hiding behind a door or concentrating on a spot on the wall) they tend to return to it over and over. Your ritual may be something to do with your personal items (hugging your pillow, biting your lavender bag, squeezing your stress ball) or it may be something you hit on at the moment of intensity. You may return to the Swirls (see page 169) for every contraction. Generally, I think women find what is most comforting in the moment.

LABOUR 'EQUIPMENT' (BIRTHING BALL, BEANBAG, ROCKING CHAIRS ETC)

If you are in a birth centre, these things may be automatically available to you, but you need to check in advance (see pages 179–81). Otherwise it may be worth investing in a few props so that you can labour for longer at home.

Birthing balls are fantastically useful for getting the baby into position during pregnancy, for sitting on if you have to work at a desk for long periods, and for 'freeing the pelvis'. They are also great as a prop for labour – if you are labouring at home in advance of going to hospital, you may find yourself sitting on it, draped over it, or even lightly bouncing on it.

Simkin also suggests cold cans of drink for pressing on your lower back as an alternative to an ice pack. I also think this is a great idea. She suggests keeping a few in the icebox in order to keep the area numb.

EMOTIONAL SUPPORT (YOUR BIRTH PARTNER)

I think Simkin is right to include the birth partner under 'natural pain relief' as the person you choose to support you in labour can be absolutely crucial to your experience of birth. (See pages 183–5 for a discussion about choosing the right birth partner.)

positions for labour

It's hard to tell in advance of labour which position you will find comfortable. You may also want to change your position as contractions intensify, or even move around. Certainly, most women agree that it is not comfortable to be restricted to a bed. While you will probably find what feels best for you naturally, below I have listed some ideas that may help.

UPRIGHT

Standing, walking, practising upright yoga positions (such as the figure-of-eight with your hips) or 'labour dancing' can be very comforting in early labour, and gravity can help labour progress.

Some attendants recommend cradling your bump from underneath and gently lifting it during a contraction to help alleviate back pain and speed up labour. Remember to bend your knees at the same time.

You can stand either supported by your partner, against a wall or holding onto something, such as the bottom of the hospital bed. Among the upright movements that you can do are Gowri Motha's 'funny walks' such as the 'elephant', 'Charlie Chaplin' and 'camel' walks, as described in her book *The Gentle Birth Method* (see page 329).

KNEELING

This can be very helpful at any time during labour, and is even a good position for giving birth. It makes it easier for your birthing attendant to check the baby's

avoid lying on your back

Lying flat on your back for any length of time late in pregnancy is not recommended. In labour it can have the effect of slowing down contractions and reducing the flow of oxygen to the baby. However, after an epidural, you will be encouraged to lie on your back, propped up by the hospital bed and pillows, or on your side because the effects of the anaesthetic can make your legs feel quite wobbly. At some hospitals you are also encouraged to give birth in this position.

heart rate and for your birth partner to apply local pressure if you are having a back labour. You can kneel in the bath or birthing pool, or in the shower with the water trained onto your back.

LEANING FORWARD

You can lean over your birthing ball, onto a beanbag, the bed, or, if he is sitting down, into a cushion on your partner's lap (also put a cushion underneath your knees). Again, this is a great position for relieving back pain and is also very comforting.

ALL FOURS

This is a wonderful position to adopt in advanced labour and, from all fours, you can practise a wide range of yoga positions. Make sure you plant your palms flat on the floor and that they are carrying most of the weight, and try not to lock your elbows. Place your knees hip-width apart. The moment you have evenly distributed your body weight, you will feel the pressure on your back and pelvis lift. You can gently rock back and forth in this position, as well as sway or outline a figure-of-eight with your hips.

THE KNEE-CHEST POSITION

If you feel your labour is progressing too quickly you can get down into the knee-chest position. Get onto all fours on some cushions and then drop your elbows to the floor so that your bottom is higher than your shoulders. Place

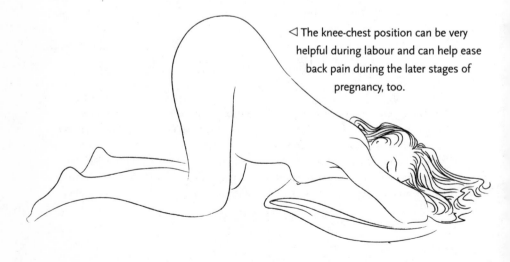

◁ The knee-chest position can be very helpful during labour and can help ease back pain during the later stages of pregnancy, too.

one wrist over the other and gently rest your head over the top. You can remain in this position for some time during a fast labour, as it allows gravity to take over and keeps the baby out of the pelvis. It can also help a posterior baby rotate and reduce the swelling of the cervix.

LYING ON YOUR SIDE
Some women like to lie on their side to concentrate on breathing in early labour, or to rest during transition. Left side is best, with a pillow between your knees.

SUPPORTED SQUATTING
This is a popular position for the second stage and can be achieved either with the support of your birth partner, a birth attendant or a birthing stool. Simply squat down and place your hands on the floor in front of you to help support your weight.

types of labour

SLOW LABOUR

First labours are often slow because the body has never been through the experience. Passageways need to stretch and the uterus needs to contract more than in subsequent labours, when the same amount of work can take less time.

There are a number of ways you can speed up a slow labour. These include:

⊙ the use of aromatherapy – clary sage is said to be particularly useful
⊙ reflexology or acupuncture – both of which use localized pressure points to speed up labour
⊙ walking around – gravity helps speed up labour
⊙ nipple stimulation – this releases oxytocin, which is needed to keep labour going
⊙ relaxing – it sounds simple and it is. For oxytocin to flow freely you need to feel relaxed, happy, safe and secure. Try listening to some music or a birthing CD, and perhaps run yourself a bath with some nice labour-stimulating oils. Escape from anyone who is making you feel uncomfortable
⊙ pelvic rocking, lunges and squatting – these can all help the baby to move into a better position and will help labour progress from within
⊙ go to sleep – while most women say that sleep couldn't have been further from their minds in a first labour, it is great for relaxation and retuning into your body. Labours can go on for days – literally – so getting some rest in early labour, when things are a bit haphazard, can be a great investment.

The average first stage in a first labour will last between 12 and 14 hours. The average second stage is between 30 minutes and two-and-a-half hours. Second and subsequent labours tend to be much shorter. Fourth- and fifth-timers can have extremely short labours.

BACK LABOUR

So called back labour often affects women whose babies are in the occipito posterior position (see page 103) and so a first recourse should be to try the movements I have suggested on pages 104 and 164 for getting the baby to move into a better position. Back labours can be drawn out, so please try to conserve your energy and rest whenever you can.

You can also help the situation by:

⊙ getting onto your hands and knees – your back will be parallel to the floor and this will encourage the baby to turn
⊙ leaning over a beanbag or birthing ball
⊙ using a hot compress on the area where you feel the pain
⊙ asking your partner to apply pressure in the painful area, either with a tennis ball or with his hands (see page 237)
⊙ remembering to keep drinking and emptying your bladder.

FAST OR 'PRECIPITATE' LABOUR

The average labour is between 15 and 16 hours for first-time mothers, seven to eight hours for second-time mothers. However, very fast labours do happen, particularly with third and fourth births and, very occasionally, a first-time labour can be very fast. This can be unpleasant, intense and extremely distressing for the mother. She has no time to build any rhythm with her body and the contractions can shift from painless to ferocious within an hour.

If you find yourself in this position, call for help in whatever way you can, by alerting someone close to you or by calling an ambulance yourself. Open the front door to allow the ambulance service a quick entry, then get into a position that you feel comfortable in or try to catch up with the intensity by getting down onto all fours with your forearms on the floor to tilt your head downwards, breathing deeply, with long out-breaths. This will help you keep calm and focused. You may find yourself moving around in an effort to find a position that works. This is fine, but try not to use any upright position as you want to slow down your labour. If the labour is highly intense or you feel the urge to poo, get into the knee-chest position (see page 242). If you need to get into a car, stay on your hands and knees in the back.

WHAT TO DO IF THE BABY COMES BEFORE THE MIDWIFE

There are plenty of stories of women giving birth in hospital car parks, in the lift on the way to the labour ward and, many years ago, I remember a husband who delivered his wife on Westminster Bridge in the back seat of the car. The thing to remember about these situations is that everything happens so fast there is usually little time to panic, and you must do what you can to stay calm. If you have someone with you, that person must keep reassuring you and tell you that you are doing well. If alone, you must try to focus mentally and tell yourself, mantra-like, that you will be okay and to stay calm. Call 999 for support as soon as physically possible so they can ensure an ambulance is called immediately. Try to give as much detail as possible and, if the baby starts to arrive before the ambulance does, they will guide you through the birth.

If you feel that the baby's head is crowning with no prior warning, open the door and get onto the floor on all fours (which helps slow things down). If things are not slowing, put your bottom in the air and your knees to your chest. Keep shouting for help. It may sound faintly ludicrous, but try to stay calm and breathe gently. If the baby is being born, pant through the stinging stretch and try not to push your baby out in one big push but in gentle pants so that your perineum has time to stretch.

Once born, hold the baby against your skin and wrap both of you in a blanket to keep warm. Don't try to get up, don't touch the cord and watch for the amount of bleeding. Wait for the ambulance to arrive.

going to the hospital

WHEN SHOULD I GO TO THE HOSPITAL?

All being well, your hospital bag should be packed, the car should be ready, or taxi or lift organized (see pages 223–4) when you want to leave. The only thing you need to think about now is making yourself as comfortable as possible in early labour. If this is your first time, you may feel anxious and excited and want to get to the hospital as soon as you feel the first contraction. Don't. Use 'patience, patience' as your mantra. By far the best place for you to spend your early labour is at home where you feel comfortable and relaxed and where labour can build up uninhibited. If you have set up your sanctuary (see pages 168–9) you can retreat there when you need to. Otherwise carry on as normal.

When your contractions build up to some regularity, call the hospital – or your midwife directly if you have her number. Midwives and doctors will usually do an over-the-phone assessment, asking questions about your labour so far, and they will probably want to speak to you during a contraction to judge the intensity.

If they decide you should come in, remember that labour can slow down or even stop altogether once you are there. Don't panic. This is just your body adjusting to the change of environment. Start putting in place all your 'snuggly bits', dim the lights and try to relax. Labour will soon start up again when you are feeling safe and relaxed and the oxytocin starts to flow again.

the initial assessment

When you arrive in hospital, your midwife will examine you. Normally there are four things she will be checking, aside from the basics of blood and urine, when she begins the examination. These are:

⊙ the lie, position and presentation of your baby
⊙ how dilated the neck of your womb has become (this is measured in centimetres from 0–10; 10 is fuly dilated and ready to push)
⊙ your baby's heart rate (see below)
⊙ the strength and frequency of your contractions.

Your midwife should also be asking you what you are thinking and how you are feeling. I personally consider this to be one of the most important questions. Don't bury any information you are unsure of, tell your medical staff exactly how you feel. This will give your midwife or doctor a deeper understanding of what is happening in your labour. It may even be the first signal of something being wrong.

THE LIE, POSITION AND PRESENTATION OF YOUR BABY

The midwife will determine this by feeling your abdomen. In a 'textbook' pregnancy, your baby's head will be head down after 36 weeks of pregnancy. That's not always the case, of course. The midwife will want to gauge:

- ⊙ how far your baby's head has descended into your pelvis
- ⊙ which way the baby's head is facing
- ⊙ if the head is 'flexed' (with his or her chin on the chest).

The occipito anterior position (see page 103) is the most straightforward presentation for delivery.

DILATION

This is a fairly rudimentary examination that involves the midwife checking your cervix with her fingers. It's better to go to the loo first – a full bladder can make the examination uncomfortable. I suggest that, during these examinations (and there may be a few in labour), you relax your mind, use visualisation techniques and relax your leg and vaginal muscles.

You can be examined in a number of positions, from standing or kneeling to squatting, but in the majority of cases you will be asked to lie down. While this position may be uncomfortable, it is the easiest and fastest way for your midwife (or obstetrician) to get the information they need.

In the early stages of labour it might make it easier still if you sit on your fists and tilt your pelvis upwards. Later on, as your cervix dilates, it may be more comfortable to sit up or even stand.

In addition to checking how open the cervix is, the midwife will assess other factors, such as the position of the baby's head, if there is caput succadameum (swelling of scalp), or moulding (overriding skull bones on the baby's head).

THE BABY'S HEART RATE

There are a few ways to measure the baby's heart rate. In low-risk cases and in home births, the heart rate can be monitored intermittently on a hand-held Doppler. In hospital there is also the option of a cardiotocograph (CTG), which is a device for recording your contractions and the foetal heart rate. It also records the relationship between your contractions and the baby's heart rate. In some cases it is used during antenatal appointments, so you may have already come across it.

A midwife will hook you up to the CTG by strapping two elastic belts around your abdomen. These hold in place two discs that are attached to the CTG with wires. The discs (transducers) record both the baby's heart rate and your contractions on graph paper (they appear as peaks and troughs), although in some hospitals they are attached to a computer.

While CTG is not considered necessary in low-risk cases, your midwife may use it if she is covering more than one labour, or when it is hospital policy. CTG monitoring does not automatically signal there is anything wrong. It is a 'screening' – as opposed to a 'diagnostic' – device. As such it has to be interpreted by your midwife or obstetrician.

If you have any concerns about the CTG or your baby's heart rate when the midwife is out of the room, get hold of someone immediately. It may just be that you have lost the trace because the transducer has moved slightly.

midwives and shift changes

Some women need a constant companion, preferably an experienced member of medical staff (or a doula) who will remain with them as long as possible. In this scenario a shift change can be very upsetting.

If the midwife you have formed a bond with suddenly clocks off and is replaced with one you don't like as much, don't panic. Remember the advice and guidance of the first midwife. If necessary, shut your eyes and keep her voice with you. You will have this baby: you can have this baby. Don't get distracted by a change of team.

You may find the shift change works to your advantage. Your midwife may change and the new midwife may be the one you form the best bond with.

However, it might also be because the baby's heart rate has dropped – and this needs urgent attention. Your baby's heart rate on the CTG can be influenced by:

⊙ the mother becoming dehydrated through vomiting or not drinking enough water
⊙ a long labour
⊙ the transducer picks up the mother's, as opposed to the baby's, heart rate.

One of the main problems with using a CTG machine is that the wires can restrict movement. You may be able to sit on a rocking chair or rock on all fours, but you won't be able to move around. Telemetry (wireless monitoring) allows you to walk freely around the labour ward or even get into a bath or birthing pool. This is particularly great for high-risk women who have to be closely monitored but want to enjoy as normal a labour as possible. Unfortunately, telemetry is not as common as it should be.

The CTG machine shouldn't dominate the labour room and, even in high-risk cases, there are ways of adapting the environment. You could, for example, ask the midwife to turn down the volume. You could also use the fact that you can see the machine plot the peaks of your contraction on paper as a mental aid to overcoming each one – the pile of paper on the floor is the journey completed and, as each contraction passes, you are one step closer to meeting your baby.

high-risk monitoring

If a mother has any pre-existing or pre-diagnosed problems (such as a previous Caesarean section or pre-eclampsia), you will automatically be monitored continuously. The same goes for a situation where there could be problems for the baby, such as when the baby is premature or has foetal growth restriction (FGR).

While I accept it is hard to hear you are 'high-risk' and not feel worried, it is also entirely possible to go on to have an incredible natural birth using dim lighting, aromatherapy massage and skin-to-skin contact. You can adapt your environment to make it as peaceful, calm and relaxing as possible. Some of the most incredible, powerful and positive labours I have witnessed have been with women categorized as high-risk (see case studies on pages 199 and 202–3).

I was recently invited by Professor Philip Bennett at Queen Charlotte's Hospital to help look after a woman who was undergoing an induction but still wanted a waterbirth. She was continuously monitored by telemetry, her syntocinon drip was powered by battery rather than the hospital electrical supply and her safety was never compromised. She had a beautiful and successful underwater birth. We normalized the abnormal.

CASE STUDY **WHEN TO SPEAK UP**

'I followed every piece of advice when I was pregnant for the first time. I went swimming every day, I went to yoga, I read pregnancy and birth books and I drank raspberry leaf tea and used lavender oil in my bath every night for the last month. I also drew up a birth plan with my partner Michael. What I didn't check in advance was how the hospital would react.

'One piece of advice I would give to a first timer would be to check your hospital's policy and view of your birth plan. Ask them whether they are going to make it difficult for you. Argue your case – you do have a choice.'

When I arrived at the hospital I was having contractions every three minutes. I was put into a brightly lit room and a seemingly endless stream of people came to check on me, strap monitors around me, prod me, examine me and question me. I didn't know that I could ask them to leave the room, dim the lights or run me a bath, so I let them take over. I had no complications, yet I was strapped to a monitor for most of the labour.

I found it most comfortable in an upright position, but the midwife told me that the monitor kept slipping, so I had to get onto the bed. In my birth plan I had stated that I didn't want to be on a bed. All my plans were unravelling and I felt I was being directed by a bunch of people I'd never met before, who apparently knew what was best for me.

Eventually a nice midwife let me go onto all fours on the bed, a kind of compromise. I felt I had reclaimed a bit of my birth, but then my contractions started to slow down. The midwives suggested that the best thing "if you don't want a slow labour" would be to break my waters, which they did. The labour then became very intense. I tried to stay on top of it, but everything was spiralling out of control.

I was still on the bed, still strapped to the monitor. The nice midwife, who was very reassuring and kept telling me I was doing well, went off and another midwife took over. She had a different approach and kept asking me if I was "finding it too hard?" I lost my nerve and before I knew it, I was having an epidural and moved to a delivery room. Everything became very clinical and tense and then a doctor came in and said, "Right, we need to get this baby out now." The whole of the pushing stage was a blur, with people looking anxious and serious and shouting instructions at me. It was awful. I ended up with an "assisted" delivery and very bad tearing.

I was very strong during my pregnancy, and in retrospect I should have stayed strong for my labour. I knew what I wanted. I didn't know I would have to fight for it. One piece of advice I would give to a first timer would be to check your hospital's policy and view of your birth plan. Ask them whether they are going to make it difficult for you. Argue your case – you do have a choice.

My second piece of advice is to prep your birth partner. If you are in labour, he or she can argue for you. That person may end up being your voice, so make sure they know what you want to say.' RACHEL, 35

the stages of labour

There are three stages of labour. Below I describe these stages, explaining what is happening to the body during each stage and giving advice on how to cope with that stage and to trust your body. The three stages of labour are as follows:

⊙ the first stage – this begins at the point at which contractions start causing the cervix to open completely. I have subdivided the first stage into smaller categories, pre-labour, active labour, advanced labour and 'transition'
⊙ the second stage – this takes over from 'transition'. It is when you have achieved full dilation and go on to push the baby out
⊙ the third stage – this is when the placenta is delivered.

the first stage

PRE-LABOUR (0–3CM DILATED)

Pre-labour or 'latent phase' describes the run up to labour, during which you may experience Braxton Hicks (see pages 91 and 138–9). The Braxton Hicks contractions are helping the baby move down into the pelvis and your cervix is shortening, opening and dilating. This part of the first stage can take a few days but, as the contractions intensify, you will know that this is the real thing. It can be a stop-start phase and even when the contractions are very strong, you still may not be experiencing 'established labour'.

The best way of coping with pre-labour is to have a positive approach to the journey as it begins. My advice is to carry on as normal to begin with, allowing the haphazard contractions to build naturally. Eat light food, even when you don't feel like it because of excitement or nausea. Drink plenty of water and vary your activities – take walks, rest, take warm baths, rest with

mantras for labour

Repeat any of the following phrases (or ask your birth partner to) that you feel might help you during birth:

⊙ 'you're going to be fine'
⊙ 'you're doing really well'
⊙ 'everything will be fine'
⊙ 'breathe, relax, release'
⊙ 'you're nearly there, keep going'
⊙ 'you're going to meet your gorgeous little baby so soon'.

a hot water bottle. If you are feeling energized but things are still moving slowly, you can always do some light exercise – perhaps swimming or yoga.

As things progress, you may want to stay closer to home and be alone or with your partner. Perhaps now is a good time to introduce the props of labour (see pages 188–94 and 238–40). Unless you are experiencing a fast labour, you can use upright labour positions that help regulate your contractions, and aromatherapy oils such as clary sage and jasmine. Remember to go to the loo often – you can ask your partner to remind you.

You may or may not want your partner present. Some women feel that it slows their labour and stops them concentrating. If you do want him there, you can ask him to help with touch techniques, such as massaging, with breathing exercises, or even get him to chat to you between contractions. You can bounce on your birthing ball or sway gently in a 'labour dance'.

When things are progressing nicely and the contractions are intensifying, you may wonder whether it is time to call the hospital or your midwife.

At around this point, I usually tell women to start thinking about 'the womb within and the womb without'. This means concentrating on the mechanisms of what is happening inside your uterus in order to explain the pain that you are feeling on the outside.

Think about the muscle fibres shortening, the uterus contracting and the baby being pushed down into the pelvis. Think about what is inside your womb – the baby in the amniotic sac, the placenta, the umbilical cord, and about how the contractions are affecting them. Think about your baby moving deeper into the pelvis and into the boney passageways of the birth canal. Think about your cervix opening and dilating. The thick muscle of the uterus is thrusting the baby forwards on the journey to meet you. On the outside, you can see your bump tightening and feel the power of the contracting uterus. It's truly amazing if you think about it.

ACTIVE LABOUR (3–5CM)

I diagnose labour as the point at which you are experiencing two or three contractions in 10 minutes and they are lasting 45–60 seconds. If you are examined at this point, you may be around 3cm dilated.

You will probably feel flushed and fairly energetic, mixed with surges of excitement and anticipation of what is to come. You may find a cold facecloth or a water spray helps at this point. Some women suck ice.

You will also notice that your breathing has changed and you will need to concentrate on keeping it slow and deep during contractions while regulating it in between contractions so that you 'get your breath back'.

As the active phase starts, you may start to find you want to move around and change positions in between contractions, focus your mind, and prepare yourself for the next wave. Partners can start taking a more active role at this point, providing support and companionship, as well as physical aid in the form of back rubs and hugs (if you want them).

It can take a while to reach 5cm, but the next stretch – from 6–9cm – is quicker, although far more intense.

CASE STUDY THE USE OF RITUALS

'I am self-employed so I had to work basically up until the day I went into labour with my first baby. Everyone kept telling me I had to prepare, and I meant to, but didn't get round to it.

When I got to the hospital, I was in agony and the only word on my lips was "epidural". It was hot, the middle of summer, and the hospital was packed. I couldn't believe that we had to sit in the waiting room before going into a labour room, then wait again before anyone came to see me.

The pain was unbelievable, my body just took over and I went into a zone. I paced the room, leant on the wall and held on to the bottom of the bed. I was following a little routine and it was making it easier to cope. I kept with the routine: pace, lean, hold the bed. My boyfriend turned the main light off and didn't really get involved. I think he went to sleep actually. My little routine made it seem as if the contractions go quicker and it helped me stay on top of the labour. I did this for maybe three or four hours – until I was eight centimetres. Then I had an epidural.

When I look back, I think it was a really good experience. I appreciate how good my body was at dealing with the contractions when I let go. Next time, I will prepare more and see how far I get under my own steam.' CHLOE, 31

ADVANCED LABOUR (6–9CM)

As the contractions become more intense, so you will draw on every aspect of what we have discussed. You may find you naturally shut down and the focus becomes more inward. I call this the 'looking-through-pink-glass time' because, like the postnatal haze, which I call 'the pink bubble', you never quite experience anything like it again in life.

I use the term 'pink glass' because, similar to the idea of 'rose-tinted spectacles', the hormones in your system and the sheer excitement of what is to come somehow power you on against all odds. It's often said that Mother Nature won't allow you to recapture the intensity of labour in the cold light of day because, if you could, you wouldn't try it again. It's so true of first labours.

This is the point at which your visualisations start to kick in. You will start finding comfort in the repetition of the visualisations, but also in any little 'rituals' (see pages 240 and 255) you find yourself performing. The 'snuggly bits', too, take central stage now, as your mind switches a gear and you start to focus on meeting the baby. Find your sequence and keep going with it.

Partners, a word to you: keep up the encouragement. Tell her how well she's doing. Many mothers want small sips of water between contractions – even more so if they are using Entonox. Lip salve is a good idea here too. Help her with these things.

If you haven't already tried the birthing pool or a warm bath, this may help things. Going into a bathroom can give you some privacy; the walls seem closer, almost womb-like, and you will feel snuggly.

Now is a good time to focus on the baby – 'the womb within'. Imagine your baby, chin flexed on chest, looking to your side and then rotating into the anterior position and looking backwards as he or she moves into the birth canal.

As you reach the end of this part of the first stage, you are going into transition, one of the most intense periods of labour.

TRANSITION

Transition takes you from 8–9cms to the second stage. It is traditionally known as the stage where most women become weepy and say, 'I can't go on' or 'I don't want to have a baby'. It's what I call 'the time in the wilderness' because women can feel lost and bewildered at this point. Women who have not had pain relief will often ask for an epidural now. Some shout and swear in transition, so partners should be pre-warned. Others totally withdraw and seem very distant. I've seen women completely retreat and go into a corner to lie down alone, almost animal-like.

You may experience a heavy show (see pages 231–2) at this point – the cervix is about to reach full dilation. Many women start to feel shivery with flu-like symptoms, and some feel nauseous. You may even vomit.

The contractions are very powerful now and usually last 60 seconds. You need maximum support from your partner. He needs to really encourage you and reassure you. You will also need to concentrate a lot on keeping your breathing focused and slowed-down – there may be a temptation to hyperventilate here. Try swaying together or having your partner stroke your arm or massage your foot.

It's also common to vocalize (see pages 239–40) at this stage, and this can be in the form of deep low noises, rather like a cow mooing. Again, this is almost a natural reflex, done to cope with the pain, and it can be very helpful. What you need to be careful of is high squeaking noises that can make you tense. If you find yourself doing this, bring your shoulders down and try to regain control of your breath using a low noise on the out-breath.

the second stage

THE URGE TO PUSH

You are now fully dilated – 10cm. The birth canal is not a straight slide, so to speak, but more like a hump. As you push, the baby descends and then needs to turn a slight corner before it reaches the exit (see diagrams, page 258). The baby will have reached the point of no return when you see a little bit of hair at the opening of the vagina. I would describe the contractions as 'very thrusting' in this phase, but the wonderful thing about the second stage is that there is a longer resting stage of three to five minutes between contractions.

I often recommend women move to all fours at this point, as it helps free pressure on the coccyx and tailbone. This position also reduces the pressure on the perineum and the baby's head can be gently born into the palm of the midwife's hand. You will probably have an idea of which position feels comfortable for labour for you (see pages 241–3).

As the baby descends, you may feel an intense pressure on your bottom. Some people describe it as needing to do a poo (others fear doing a poo). The urge to push at this point can be overwhelming. The baby powers down through this last bit, the chin pressing further onto the chest and the boney plates of the head overlapping to help the passage through the narrow canal.

I often get women to reach down and feel the baby's head to encourage them for the final few thrusts. Some women find it helpful to have a mirror in place to see what is happening, but most prefer to keep their eyes shut.

Just before your baby is born, the head must negotiate a 'u-bend' in the vagina and rocks up and down with contractions, disappearing from sight until the widest part of the baby's head 'crowns' and becomes visible again. As you reach this point of no return, you will experience a strong stinging sensation. This is a huge encouragement, despite the pain, as you know that it means your baby is just about to be born. I always recommend women pant or blow at this point as the head is being delivered. As if emerging through the neck of a polo neck jersey, the little forehead, then eyes, then nose, then mouth, then chin appear, until all the head is out. The baby then rotates so that the shoulders are in line with the back, which is still within the birth canal. With the next push the shoulders are born, and then the rest of the body follows. This is the point at which the time of birth is recorded and the baby is passed to you, with the cord still attached and pulsating, so you can have skin-to-skin contact, if you want it.

The time of birth is announced when the baby is completely free of the mother. The cord will pulsate for a few minutes before being clamped and cut – usually by the father or mother – with guidance from the midwife.

The baby's head may be wrinkled and swollen from the journey but this settles within 24 hours of birth.

positions for birth

Choices of birth position are important and you should be allowed, within reason, to give birth in the position that comes naturally and that you feel most comfortable in. Some women choose a conventional position, others go for a more active approach, using upright positions that enlist the powers of gravity, for example. Common positions for birth are:

⊙ the conventional position (lying on a bed or mat)
⊙ lithotomy (on your back with your legs in the air)
⊙ squatting (with or without support)
⊙ kneeling and leaning forward
⊙ sitting on a birth stool
⊙ getting down onto all fours.

how the head emerges

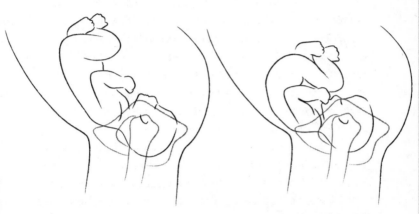

1 The baby powers down through the birth canal, its head just visible through the vaginal opening.

2 The head rocks away from the opening slightly to negotiate a slight U-bend in the vagina.

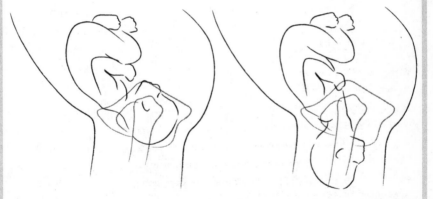

3 Past the U-bend now, the widest part of the head 'crowns', stretching the vaginal opening wide open. The mother experiences a sharp stinging sensation that accompanies this stretch.

4 As if emerging from a polo neck jersey, the forehead, then eyes, then nose, then mouth, then chin appear until the head is out. With the next push, the shoulders will emerge and the baby will be born.

the third stage

The third stage is the delivery of the placenta, which can be done either 'actively' or naturally.

If you choose an 'active' third stage, then there is no physical effort involved. You will be given an injection of either syntometrine or syntocinon in the thigh between two and seven minutes after the birth, which causes the uterus to contract again. Your midwife or doctor will simultaneously place their hand on your abdomen and, by pushing upwards while looping the cord around with the other hand and gently pulling downwards, detach the placenta from the uterine wall inside. In most cases it comes away easily and is delivered.

If you choose a natural or 'physiological' third stage, then you will deliver the placenta naturally, usually up to an hour after the baby is born. I find most women are so preoccupied with the baby they don't focus too much on the actual delivery of the placenta. Anyway, you'll be pleased to know that it is much easier than the birth of the baby.

I recommend, if you can, that you start breastfeeding immediately, as this triggers a release of oxytocin, the hormone that causes the uterus to contract again, and thus the placenta to separate from the wall of the uterus.

Your uterus will rise in response to the placenta separating, and you may experience some bleeding and the cord dropping. Sometimes I get women to sit on the loo and hold their tummy tight with both hands. This, along with gravity, will help the placenta out in the easiest way. If it drops in the loo, obviously don't flush it! The midwife will check it is intact and feel your uterus to ensure Mother Nature has done her job properly.

born in the caul

When a baby is born with the amniotic sac intact, it is called being born in the caul. I call them 'babies born with veils over them'. This is very rare – perhaps only 1 in 1,000 babies will be born in a caul. I have seen five in my career, two of which were underwater births, and the first time it took me totally by surprise.

The amniotic sac needs to be peeled off the baby by either the midwives or the mother, so that the baby can breathe.

tears and episiotomies

TEARS AND THE MEANING OF 'DEGREES'

As many as 85% of women have some perineal damage after a vaginal delivery, and 60–70% require stitches. The majority of these tears are into the perineum, and in some ways it is not surprising, given what your body has just experienced. If you haven't had an epidural, the stitches will be performed under local anaesthetic and, in most cases, they are performed in a matter of minutes. Perineal tears are most likely to occur with:

⊙ big babies, especially if they weigh over 4kg (around 8.8lbs)
⊙ instrumental or assisted deliveries, such as forceps or ventouse
⊙ babies who are born in the occipito posterior position (see page 103), looking up or 'stargazing'
⊙ babies whose shoulders get stuck (shoulder dystocia).

There is little you can do to prevent a tear. Some women swear by perineal massage (see pages 144–5), but I personally don't believe that perineal massage performed during labour itself has any effect.

Tears are defined into four degrees:
⊙ first – you have only torn the perineal or vaginal skin
⊙ second – the tear involves the posterior vaginal wall, perineal muscle and the skin
⊙ third – the tear extends to the anal sphincter, but the rectal mucosa (inner lining) is intact
⊙ fourth – the anal canal is opened and the tear may spread up along the rectum.

Although many women complain that the area 'doesn't look quite the same', in most cases the tear heals with no long-term damage or consequence and it functions as before. Some women do, however, need follow-up treatment in the form of surgery or physiotherapy.

If you have any concerns, don't be embarrassed to ask about the area – plenty of women do, particularly when it comes to postnatal sex. The key thing to remember is: pelvic floor exercises. Now you know about them, you may as well introduce them for life.

PREVENTING A TEAR

Control is essential to prevent tearing, but very difficult to enforce once you are in the throes of birth and thinking more about getting the baby out than whether you will tear. For this reason, I would say control is in the hands of the midwife. In a situation where I think there may be a bad tear I try to do the breathing out with the mother as I can see where the baby is. In this way I can direct the birth by showing her myself the way I want her to breathe.

I particularly recommend the advice of the Hypnobirthers who recommend gentle 'J breaths' as a way of 'breathing the baby out', rather than pushing. Mothers that follow this advice are far less likely to tear. For some reason, perhaps because the mother is more relaxed, home births do appear to have higher 'intact' rates.

SORENESS

You may be experiencing some perineal soreness, even if you didn't experience a tear. This is the stinging or bruised feeling that women get around the vagina and in the area between the vagina and rectum. To be frank, it's caused by pushing a baby through passageways that are usually quite small and have been forced to distend to the extreme.

WHAT HELPS? Try the following:

- ⊙ frozen preparations: if the whole area is very swollen, ice packs can bring immediate relief, although don't put ice directly onto the skin. You can use gel pads cooled in the freezer, a bag of peas in a tea towel or ice cubes in a small plastic bag wrapped in cloth – perhaps a muslin – pressed onto the area
- ⊙ anaesthetic cream or gels: these include lignocaine or lidocaine and can be topically applied
- ⊙ arnica: the medically approved homeopathic remedy. You can take this in tablet form immediately after birth and for two weeks following birth. It also comes in the form of a cream for bruises
- ⊙ witch hazel pads: again these can be used directly on the area

- pain relief: you can take tablets for both the pain and the swelling – check with your midwife what is best for you, especially if you are breastfeeding. You can also be prescribed suppositories
- pass urine regularly – a full bladder can exacerbate the pain
- move your bowels – many women have trouble doing their first poo after birth. My advice is to hold a sanitary pad at the front when you first go so that you feel supported and confident. If you are having trouble going, eat foods – such as prunes and sweetcorn – that help. Otherwise try a gentle laxative such as lactulose
- strong painkillers – such as voltoral and co-dyromol – over the initial few days (although the latter can cause constipation).

EPISIOTOMY

An episiotomy is performed when there is a danger of a tear being so bad that it goes into the rectum (back passage). You will be asked to give your consent before the procedure is carried out and it will only be done in order to prevent worse damage being done.

My view is that episiotomy should only be performed when absolutely necessary and I very rarely need to do them in spontaneous vaginal births. Around 15–17% of women in the UK have an episiotomy, but the statistics differ depending on the type of birth. You are slightly more likely to have one in a first birth (20%), and far less likely in a second birth (5%). They are used in 76% of forceps births and 58% of ventouse births. Other situations where you may need an episiotomy include:

- when delivering a big baby
- when the baby's shoulders are stuck (shoulder dystocia)
- when the baby is breech
- if you have had previous third degree tears.

The wound needs to be looked after as it is a fairly deep cut, usually involving perineal muscle. It will take a little longer to heal and evidence shows that it is more painful than a natural tear.

expecting the unexpected

Your labour journey may change direction if your baby becomes stuck or unhappy, so plan for all possible deviations from your ideal birth plan, be flexible and positive, and think of what you can still have in your labour rather than what is not possible. The most important thing is a safe baby and a safe mother.

induction of labour

Around 20% of labours in Britain are induced (artificially kick-started), according to Department of Health figures. The numbers of women who are induced have crept up annually. According to Department of Health statistics, in 2005–6, the percentage of women induced on the NHS had reached 20.2% (from 19.6% in 2004–5). Induction is the most common reason for women to deviate from their birth plans.

There are measures you can take to try and bring on labour naturally (see pages 228–9). However, in some cases you may not have the luxury of waiting to see if a natural induction works. In others, you may have tried everything and still be proceeding towards a medical induction.

Check your hospital's policy to find out if and when you may be induced. Policies change from hospital to hospital and depend on whether you are NHS or private. They will also take into account your age, previous pregnancies and other factors in your medical history.

While you may feel that you've had enough of the pregnancy and want to be induced, induction can completely change the course of a labour. Statistically, you are more likely to end up with a managed and 'medicalized' birth and pain relief. I explain to women that induction is like a little row of dominoes; once you set the first one off you trigger a chain. It's worth knowing that labours that are induced have a one-in-three-chance of ending up as emergency Caesareans.

On the other hand, you may be fiercely against induction, but are asked to consider it by your midwife and obstetrician because of your situation. You need to weigh up your options. Consider the following issues:

⊙ why does your obstetrician want you to be induced?
⊙ what are your misgivings?
⊙ which option is safer for your baby?
⊙ can you talk through the idea of waiting longer with your doctor?
⊙ is there a compromise that can be reached – e.g. if you haven't gone into spontaneous labour in, say, two days, then you will agree to be induced?

I AM LOW-RISK; FOR WHAT REASON WOULD I BE INDUCED?
NICE (the National Institute of Clinical Excellence) recommends that anyone

whose pregnancy has gone more than 41 weeks should be offered an induction. This is because, statistically, the baby is at a slightly increased risk of health problems after that date. Babies that are 'post-mature' (past 42 weeks' gestation) are at a slightly increased risk of being stillborn[18] because of placental insufficiency.

Obviously, you have some say in the matter and the decision-making should be collaborative. A mother should remain centre stage when it comes to decision-making: it is her body and her baby.

If you choose not to be induced at 41 weeks, you will be offered twice weekly checks of the baby's heart rate and an ultrasound to establish the amount of amniotic fluid around the baby from 42 weeks.

If you are uncertain what to do and are not happy to be induced, seek advice. If you feel your obstetrician or midwives are not being supportive, you can contact the Association for Improvements in the Maternity Services (see page 327 for their website address).

WHAT IS THE PROCEDURE FOR AN INDUCTION?

The decision to induce is based on if the baby and/or mother is considered safer out then remaining in the womb, and the decision is discussed between yourself and your obstetrician.

There are three components involved in induction: prostaglandin, ARM and syntocinon. In first births, all three are usually necessary. However, with subsequent births, the process may require only one or two components.

Prior to the procedure, you will pass urine, then lie down with your fists beneath your bottom (to tilt your pelvis forwards) and the soles of your feet together. Relax your thigh and vaginal muscles to make it easier for the midwife or obstetrician to find your cervix and reduce discomfort for you. Occasionally, women can find this too uncomfortable. If this is the case, you can use Entonox to help you relax.

A prostaglandin pessary or gell will be placed behind your cervix. Following insertion you will need to stay in bed for one hour to keep the pessary or gel in place, so that it can be absorbed by the area around your cervix, making it soft and thin. Your baby's heartbeat will be monitored by CTG prior to and following insertion.

When your cervix is open, the midwife or obstetrician will perform an amniotomy (or ARM – artificial rupture of the membranes) – your waters will be broken. This procedure involves a vaginal examination and the brief insertion of a thin plastic stick with a tiny sharp hook at the end. At the height of a contraction the membranes bulge and the midwife or obstetrician will make a tiny hole, allowing the amniotic fluid to flow out. Once the waters are ruptured, labour can become more intense, due to the baby's head pressing directly onto the cervix rather than being cushioned by a bag of water. The moment the water is released you will experience a strange sensation of warm water releasing. In some cases it's a rush of water, in others, simply a trickle. (An ARM can also be performed in labour if there are concerns about your baby's heartbeat or if progess is very slow. If meconium is seen in the waters you will need close monitoring of your baby's heartbeat.)

More often than not, first-time mothers need syntocinon to establish contractions. The amount of syntocinon is increased slowly until there are four contractions in every 10 minutes. A midwife or obstetrician will give you an intravenous infusion and you will be hooked up to a CTG monitor so that the baby's heart rate can be monitored to watch the baby's reaction to the contraction and ensure relaxation of contractions occur, as too much syntocinon can affect the health of your baby.

Some women who are not having any contractions prior to having the syntocinon may decide to have an epidural in advance, while others prefer a 'wait and see' approach.

assisted delivery

The most common problems encountered by babies in labour can be boiled down to two broad reasons: the heart rate showing abnormalities, or the baby getting stuck as she tries to negotiate and descend through the passageways.

There are many reasons for the head not progressing properly through the birth canal – perhaps the cervix has not opened enough, perhaps the baby's head has jammed against the middle bones of the pelvis. Or perhaps the baby is simply too big. In these scenarios you will have what is called an 'assisted delivery' – one using a ventouse machine or forceps, or an emergency Caesarean section.

Your midwife or obstetrician will advise which is the best in your case. The decision will usually be based on the extent to which the neck of the womb has opened and how low the baby's head has descended.

You will also be given a Caesarean if the neck of the womb is part closed and either the labour is not progressing, or the baby is unhappy (which your midwife will be able to tell from the heart rate).

EPISIOTOMY

Around 15–17% of women in the UK have an episiotomy and you are more likely to be given one if you are having an assisted delivery. An episiotomy is a surgical incision, usually 1–2cm in length at the vaginal opening, either on the perineum or to the side of it (see also page 263). This increases the size of the opening to allow the baby to pass through more easily. The procedure is favoured over natural tearing only when it is thought that the damage will be worse without one. Unfortunately an episiotomy cut takes longer to heal and causes far more pain than a natural tear.

An episiotomy might be used in the event of a:

⊙ ventouse delivery: it is commonly used in ventouse deliveries, but not always. An experienced practitioner will be able to judge whether or not it is appropriate
⊙ forceps delivery: an episiotomy is always used with forceps deliveries because the vaginal opening is distended by the blades of the forceps
⊙ shoulder dystocia (when the baby's shoulders are stuck): in this case the

obstetrician or midwife needs to widen the opening to make more space so that they can manually rotate the baby or bring down the posterior arm

⊙ breech presentation: you may be given an episiotomy for a breech birth in order to protect the baby's head, but it is not a given

⊙ premature births

⊙ third or fourth degree tears (because there is a danger that the tear will go into the rectum)

⊙ big baby

⊙ baby that is in the direct occipito posterior presentation (see page 103), so the diameter of the head coming down over the perineum is 13.5cm as opposed to 9.5cm.

For advice on how to treat a sore perineum after an episiotomy or tearing, see pages 262–3.

VENTOUSE

Both ventouse and forceps deliveries are usually performed by an obstetrician. The obstetrician will first touch your abdomen to establish how low the baby's head has descended. If the baby's head is more than 'one fifth palpable' (more than one fifth of it can be felt by a midwife when feeling or 'palpating' the abdomen), he or she will usually perform a Caesarean section.

There is more than one type of ventouse and it is only used for women in the second stage of labour (the pushing stage), when the baby's head is low.

Nearly 11% of babies born in the UK are 'instrumental delivery', (ventouse or forceps), according to Department of Health statistics for 2004–5. The likelihood of having an 'instrumental delivery' drops dramatically if you are a second-time mother.

So, when are you likely to have a ventouse? Well, you may have been through a very long and even very successful first stage but, by the time you get to the second stage, you may be feeling exhausted. Medical staff may suggest a ventouse if:

⊙ your baby's heart rate has dropped and the obstetrician is called

⊙ your baby is distressed

⊙ you are very tired

⊙ you are finding it hard to summon up the strength to push hard enough

- ⊙ tissues on the perineum do not stretch easily
- ⊙ you are distressed and just can't take it anymore
- ⊙ you have high blood pressure
- ⊙ you have cardiac disease and your heart cannot cope with the exertion of pushing in the second stage.

Women have a mixed response to this: some feel relief, some disappointment. Remember, the aim is to get the safest outcome for mother and child and it's important to feel positive about that.

So let's imagine you've been told you need a ventouse delivery. What happens next? The obstetrician has arrived. First he or she will carry out a vaginal examination. You may then be placed in the lithotomy position (lying on your back with your bottom positioned at the end of the bed and your feet in stirrups). The bottom of your bed will be removed and then the bed will be raised so that the doctor can get in the best position for easing the baby out of the birth canal.

They will establish which way the baby's head is facing in the pelvis, which will determine the best place to attach the ventouse cup. Once they are sure there are no parts of vaginal tissue under the cup, the midwife will turn on the suction machine. First on a low setting, then gradually increased.

The ventouse is a push–pull procedure. As soon as the next contraction arrives, you push down and the doctor pulls and guides the baby's head around the birth canal. Usually the baby's head will be born after two to three pushes. Occasionally the cup can slip off, perhaps because the baby has too much hair to achieve a proper suction attachment, or if the baby's scalp is too swollen for successful attachment.

Ventouse is still the instrument of choice for an instrumental delivery. The Royal College of Obstetricians and Gynaecologists (RCOG) Green-top Guidelines recommend ventouse over forceps wherever possible. There are good reasons for this – it is easier to use, the baby is less likely to be bruised as a result and you are less likely to tear your perineum (many women don't even need stitches).

Don't forget that once your baby is born and in your arms you can revert to your Utopia birth plan. All being well, you can enjoy your skin-to-skin bonding and the 'magical moments' of birth.

KIWI VENTOUSE

The kiwi ventouse is a small hand-held device which has a suction cup attached. It achieves suction by the obsetrician squeezing the device. Unlike the traditional ventouse, it does not need to be attached to a larger electrical machine to achieve suction.

The benefits of this small device are that it is easily transported, easily used, not frightening to look at and, in some units, can be used by midwives. The disadvantage is that it may not be as successful in helping women to achieve a vaginal birth as the conventional ventouse because it does not provide as much suction. Sometimes the suction cup detaches. There are no differences between the two types of ventouse in terms of injury to mother or baby.

When talking to your midwife and obstetrician about ventouse, ask if there is a choice between kiwi ventouse or conventional, as some units may have one or other, some may use both types. If the kiwi omnicup does not work as a first measure, you may find that a forceps delivery is recommended.

FORCEPS DELIVERY

Forceps deliveries are needed if your baby needs to be 'lifted out' of the pelvis. The baby should be born with two pulls. The procedure begins with you being placed in the lithotomy position (lying on your back with your bottom positioned at the end of the bed and your feet in stirrups). Forceps delivery requires an episiotomy.

So what do forceps look like? Strangely enough, they look like an enormous pair of salad servers. They lock together around the baby's head and allow the doctor to both support the head and guide it around the curve of the birth canal.

Forceps babies are often born with a little bruising on their heads, and even marks on each side of the face caused by the instrument. Both the bruising and the marks should subside within a couple of days.

With both ventouse and forceps, I strongly advise that the baby receives Vitamin K intramuscularly as opposed to orally (in the mouth) to help with any clotting.

In both these types of delivery you can put a hand down if you want to feel your baby's head coming out and you can ask to see your baby emerging by putting the top of the bed up more.

I would go as far as to say that it is important to have skin-to-skin contact with your baby as soon as possible in this scenario so that no magic moments are missed. I am an advocate of delaying the cutting of the umbilical cord, where possible, and if the baby is 37 weeks or more and crying immediately, there should be no reason why he shouldn't be delivered straight into your arms.

Otherwise, the resuscitaire should be in the delivery room alongside you and a paediatrician is normally present.

emergency Caesarean

An emergency Caesarean is one that needs to take place as quickly as possible in order to keep mother, baby, or both as safe as possible. Once the obstetrician has made a decision to operate, it is recommended that the baby should be born within 30 minutes. A very important point to remember if you find yourself in a situation where you have to have an emergency Caesarean is that many women have managed to stay positive and had a great outcome even after an emergency Caesarean. One example I can share was the case of a very fit yoga teacher who was having her first baby at home.

The baby initially made very good progress and, in quite a short number of hours, the mother was 6cm dilated. However, at around that point the baby got 'stuck' in the mid-pelvis and she didn't dilate any further. The mother was in the pool and we were talking throughout the labour. I was actually surprised that the cervix wasn't dilating further, and a little baffled. I could only imagine that the baby was bigger than we'd all previously thought.

Finally, I decided a transfer to hospital was necessary. The mother agreed. Pretty quickly the hospital staff and I realized that there was no option but an emergency Caesarean and she was whisked straight into theatre.

When the baby arrived she weighed just under 11lb (5kg). The average baby girl born at term weighs 7.6lb (3.45kg). No one could believe it. I was so relieved that we had done a Caesarean section – and so was the mother. She described it as a 'wonderful birth' despite the massive detour in her birth plan.

reasons for an emergency Caesarean

Emergency Caesareans usually take place after labour has already started. In some cases – such as an illness or an accident that endangers the baby's life, or a placenta abruption (when the placenta detaches from the uterine wall), an emergency Caesarean will be performed before labour commences.

FAILURE TO PROGRESS
Failure to progress (FTP) means that, although you are in labour, your cervix is

not opening at a rate considered safe, or that the baby is 'stuck'. There can be a number of reasons for why the baby can get stuck in a first labour:

- the passageways have never been stretched in this way before and the abdominal muscle is strong
- your cervix isn't opening. This can be a soft-tissue problem. There is also evidence to show that this is more likely to happen to women who have had surgery in this area. For example, a loop excision can create fibrous tissues that don't stretch well and, as a result, the cervix fails to stretch
- the baby is positioned badly as he descends into the pelvis. For example, if his chin is not tucked under, the circumference of the head is much greater, making it harder for him to pass through the birth canal. Your baby is also more likely to get stuck if he is in the occipito posterior position (see page 103)
- your baby is an 'undiagnosed breech'
- your baby shows 'distress' – this will be picked up if there are dramatic changes in the baby's heart rate. Distress can be caused by a number of reasons: the cord is around the baby's neck; there are twists in the cord; the amniotic fluid around the baby may be depleted, which means there is less cushioning around the baby; the placenta is not functioning well
- your baby passes meconium in the waters – which can also be a sign of distress. In this case, medical staff may fear that the toxic meconium could get into the baby's lungs. Again, it can also be a sign that the placenta hasn't been working properly
- the baby is very big. Usually big babies are diagnosed in advance of labour during your antenatal check up. Your midwife or doctor will 'palpate' (feel) your abdomen and check the 'height of fundus' with a tape measure. If there are any concerns about the baby's size, she will refer you for an ultrasound. In this way, the doctor can also check the amount of amniotic fluid around a baby as well as the size. If the baby is on the 97th percentile, you will probably be offered the option of a Caesarean section, but the obstetrician will go through the pros and cons with you before you make a decision.

what happens?

If you are rushed for an emergency Caesarean, the pre-op procedure will include you being hooked up to an intravenous infusion. You will be monitored by CTG and the upper part of the pubic hairline will be shaved. Unless you have passed urine recently, you will be fitted with a catheter. As you will have already had the epidural, this shouldn't hurt. An anaesthetist will then assess you. Your epidural may be topped up or you may be given a pudendal nerve block that numbs the tissues around the vagina. You can ask for your own music (although I wouldn't recommend anything too hypnotic – you don't want the team affected).

The doctor will be 'scrubbing in', putting on a sterile gown and opening a sterile 'delivery pack'. Drapes – usually made of paper – will be placed on your abdomen and then over each leg, a bit like the sleeves of a very big jersey. The obstetrician will then put a sheet under your bottom so that only the area for delivery is left exposed. He or she will then re-examine you vaginally to check your cervix and the position of your baby. At this point he will decide whether he could use the ventouse or the forceps instead of performing a Caesarean. You should always, always, be kept informed of his decisions.

If he decides to continue with the operation he will inform the other staff. For a Caesarean section there will be at least eight people in the room with you:

⊙ the anaesthetist
⊙ the anaesthetic nurse
⊙ the obstetric surgeons performing the operation
⊙ the obstetric surgeon assisting
⊙ a neonatal doctor
⊙ a midwife
⊙ a scrub nurse
⊙ a 'circulating nurse' to assist the scrub nurse.

As I've said when discussing the 'natural Caesarean' (see pages 207–9), at Queen Charlotte's we have the drape down so mothers don't miss out on any magic moments of birth. They see the baby's head emerge, followed by the arms, the body, then the legs. The doctor cuts the cord and then either he or the midwife hands the baby to the mother. You can enjoy skin-to-skin contact and I have seen babies breastfeeding while their mothers were being sutured.

crashing emergencies

Now we come to the bit where you may think it would be hard to stay positive. A crash Caesarean is one where the baby must come out as quickly as possible in order to save the baby's or mother's life, in cases where there is cord prolapse, the baby's heart rate is abnormally low, or severe pre-eclampsia, for example. Often there is no time for an epidural so a general anaesthetic will be given.

It is very important for everyone to remain calm and for someone to be with you at all times. It can be terrifying to arrive in a hospital in an emergency, or to be transferred in an emergency situation.

The medical team may not have time to talk things through with you as normal, as a crashing emergency requires clear decisive action. Women have described it as a very lonely experience, but try to hold on to the knowledge that the team's primary concern is you and your baby. They will act as quickly as possible to keep you safe.

Operating theatres are set up to cope with emergencies. Everything, from the equipment to the doctors, will be ready. Other departments, such as the neo-natal intensive care unit for premature babies, will be put on standby. A sea of medical staff will be busying around you and it is quite normal to feel like you are going through some kind of out-of-body or dream-like experience. If you have lost a lot of blood, you may also feel faint. It's okay to communicate how you are feeling while, at the same time, letting the team get on with their work. The calmer you all are, the easier it is to take control of the emergency.

If your situation requires a lot of medical attention, you may be put under general anaesthetic. Don't lose hope of clawing back something from your birth plan. Anything your partner and family can do to help reduce anxiety and care for you psychologically will greatly help your recovery. I remember one lady I cared for suffered a massive haemorrhage shortly after giving birth. After the surgery, she reverted to the birth she'd always wanted – she held her beautiful little baby skin-to-skin. While she was under the anaesthetic her husband had held the baby skin-to-skin and then related all these moments to her when she came round.

premature birth

If you go into labour at any time between 20 and 37 weeks your baby will be premature or 'preterm'. Premature babies, particularly those born before 28 weeks can suffer significant long-term problems. Around 7% of babies are premature in the UK – that is 45,000 out of 650,000.

Premature birth is an area that still requires much research. While obstetricians can put in place a number of precautions to stop a premature birth reoccurring in a second or subsequent pregnancy, they often don't know why it happened in the first place. Half of all premature babies are born after an unexplained spontaneous labour with no apparent 'risk factors'.

WHAT WOULD PUT ME AT RISK OF A PREMATURE LABOUR?

If you are affected by any of the following, there is a risk of premature labour:

⊙ high blood pressure, and the associated risk of pre-eclampsia
⊙ a multiple pregnancy – which can overstretch the womb
⊙ diabetes
⊙ obstetric cholestasis
⊙ previous gynaecological surgery, which may have caused damage to the neck of the womb
⊙ lifestyle factors such as drinking too much alcohol, smoking, recreational drugs, excess caffeine, poor diet or eating disorders (being underweight)
⊙ an incompetent cervix
⊙ problems with the placenta – for example, if the placental blood supply is impaired, if it detaches from the uterine wall (placenta abruption) or if the placenta is 'calcified'
⊙ infection – of either the bladder or vagina
⊙ damage to the amniotic sac
⊙ urinary or vaginal infection. If you suspect that you have any urine or vaginal infection, you need to report it as soon as possible.

PREMATURE LABOUR

The most obvious symptom of premature labour is painful contractions, but it may be that your waters break early. When you arrive at hospital, you will be asked to describe what has been happening. The staff will ask you questions such as:

⊙ how long have your contractions been coming?
⊙ how many minutes have lapsed between contractions?
⊙ have you experienced any bleeding?
⊙ have your waters broken, or have you experienced any fluid loss, no matter how small?
⊙ have you had a previous preterm baby?
⊙ have you had any previous infections?
⊙ do you smoke, drink or take recreational drugs?

If your waters haven't broken, you will be examined internally to see how dilated you are. The doctor will also take a swab to see if you have an infection.

If you are between 22–23 weeks pregnant, you may have what is called a 'fibronectin assessment' – if the presence of fibronectin is detected it may indicate that labour has started.

Fortunately, most (that is, 60% of) women who experience preterm contractions find the labour settles down and they go on to full term. For the remaining 40%, labour will continue and you will be transferred to a specialized unit, if possible, before the baby is delivered. You will probably be given an intravenous tocolytic drug that lessens the contractions and slows the labour. This creates valuable time that can be used both for artificially maturing the baby's lungs with steroids and transferring the mother to a hospital with neonatal facilities.

If the baby is 'head down' then he or she can be delivered vaginally. If the baby is breech, he or she will be delivered by Caesarean section.

A premature baby's survival rate is determined by how many weeks you are when you deliver. If you are 30 weeks plus, your baby has a very good chance of a good recovery with no long-term effects. A baby born before 24 weeks has a 50% risk of disability.

NEONATAL CARE UNIT
Most of us do not expect to find our babies in neonatal units and, unfortunately, nothing anyone can say can prepare parents for the shock. Your baby will be attached to monitoring equipment – particularly breathing support – and may

require repeated injections in his or her very tiny veins. This can be extremely upsetting and you will need a lot of support from friends and family as well as the medical team at your hospital.

There are three different levels of care:

⊙ intensive care (also called NICU), for the most seriously ill preterm babies
⊙ high-dependency care, for those who are not critical but need complex care
⊙ special care, for premature babies who are catching up on growth.

'KANGAROO CARE' Paediatricians recommend 'kangaroo care' for premature babies as soon as possible, which basically means holding your tiny baby next to your naked skin. This idea was originated in 1983 when two Colombian doctors, Neos Edgar Rey and Hector Martinez, introduced the idea in a desperate effort to bring down the high mortality rate among premature babies. Their findings have been taken up all over the world and are now commonplace in all neonatal units in the UK and on mainstream labour wards with term babies. See page 282 for more on this.

A more recent Canadian study of premature babies born between 28 and 32 weeks showed how those given blood tests while being held skin-to-skin at their mother's breast seemed to experience less pain than those who had blood samples taken while lying in the cot.

meeting your baby

The moment when you meet your baby is charged with emotions. Your baby is placed in your arms, or skin-to-skin on your chest and you touch your baby with tenderness, whispering words of love. The light is subdued and slowly, your baby opens her eyes wide. Take mental pictures of the experience to keep with you forever.

bonding with your baby

MAGICAL MOMENTS

The birth is over, your midwife passes you your baby and, suddenly, you are catapulted into motherhood. It may have felt like forever for this treasured moment to arrive. Throughout pregnancy, questions may have played on your mind. Is my baby all right? What will he or she look like? Will I be a good mother? What will our first moments face-to-face be like?

Now you are here, you will be experiencing a mixture of emotions – perhaps exhaustion, relief, exhilaration and amazement. The baby is squirming in your arms, vernix smeared and with soggy hair, all squashed and extraordinary, smelling delicious. You can finally look into her grey-black eyes that, until now, have only known the darkness of the womb. After a few moments of adjustment to the light, your baby can also look back at you.

I call these the 'falling in love moments', the 'I can't believe you are my baby' moments. These are wonderful moments in the miracle of birth. Your baby may remain in the foetal position, not immediately aware that the walls of the womb are no longer hugging her. Slowly she may stretch and experiment with her new surroundings. Although the place is strange, there is the comforting and familiar smell of her mother next to her.

She can lie on your skin, feel the vibrations of your heartbeat and hear your voice – the voice she has come to know. This is her 'womb without', a place she can be protected, loved and nurtured on the outside.

Try to savour these moments for as long as possible, without the humdrum of hospital procedure crashing into your sanctuary. You may even be experiencing these moments after a delay because of an emergency procedure. Perhaps you have been through huge surges of emotion after a difficult birth.

I recommend that, however and wherever your baby is born, you claw back these important moments. If you are separated from your baby at birth you could always ask for something of yours to be kept with her, a 'snuggly bit', if you like, perhaps a scarf or T-shirt.

If you are in the operating theatre, the baby may spend her first skin-to-skin time with Dad. If baby and Mum need assistance, perhaps ask the father to take digital photographs so that you can look at her while you wait for your 'magical moments' together. Once you and your baby feel well enough, you can be reunited and enjoy these first moments together as much as if they had happened straight after birth. They are still your 'falling in love' moments, no matter when they happen.

THE BEAUTY OF SKIN-TO-SKIN CONTACT

The idea of skin-to-skin contact originated in Bogota in Colombia in 1983, as a way of helping premature babies thrive. Two doctors discovered that babies that had 'kangaroo care' (see page 279) had better survival rates. Their findings were adopted elsewhere and follow-up studies found that all babies benefited from immediate skin-to-skin contact for up to an hour after birth. Research published in 2003[19] showed the effects of the practice on healthy babies born at term.

The review covered 30 studies, surveying a total of 1,925 new mothers and their babies. It found that, after a period of skin-to-skin:

- interaction with the mother was greater
- babies stayed warmer
- babies cried less
- mothers breastfed for longer
- babies breastfed more easily
- babies' heart rates were more stable.

As there are no reported adverse reactions to skin-to-skin contact, only benefits, there is no harm in doing it for as long and as often as possible, if your baby is well enough. And it doesn't have to just be skin-to-skin with the mother. The father can play this role, too. A recent Swedish study showed that skin-to-skin with fathers when mothers still needed medical assistance promoted the same calming and comforting effects as with the mother.

In an ideal world, I would like British hospitals to follow the example of Sweden, where all babies enjoy one hour of skin-to-skin (if well enough) after birth. The benefits are significant. It means that midwives, obstetricians and paediatricians need to adapt the speed of their routines and rituals post birth, and allow the mother and baby that time together.

WHAT IF I'M TOO EXHAUSTED TO HOLD MY BABY IMMEDIATELY?

Obviously skin-to-skin is fabulous, but there are many mothers – especially first timers – who are too stunned, too exhausted or, to be frank, in too much pain for immediate skin-to-skin. If you find yourself in this situation, don't worry and don't feel guilty. It's very common to feel in shock after birth. This is where sometimes quite animated women will suddenly go quiet and shut down. Their eyes will zone out and they may appear to be in a daze. You may feel sick, bewildered, faint or just 'out of it'. You may have lost blood and need drugs and fluids, or need extensive stitching.

It's completely normal to need time to recover – the marathon of labour is a hugely emotional and physical journey and everyone responds to it differently. This may well mean that you can't immediately hold your little baby. Usually this is a good time for partners to step in and take over with the little one, perhaps doing a bit of skin-to-skin and keeping him or her warm, while the mother is given time to collect herself and feel better.

WHAT IF I DON'T FEEL AN IMMEDIATE BOND WITH MY BABY?
DON'T WORRY. Many, many first-time mums feel completely shell-shocked by the experience of birth and the sudden realization that they have a new baby. This can temporarily interrupt the immediate bonding process that you may have with second or subsequent children, but it is entirely normal and not something to worry about.

Women often say that they knew their baby when it was wriggling and kicking inside, but they are suddenly confronted with a stranger when it arrives. 'I looked at the baby and saw three generations of different family members in this one little original face,' one mother told me. 'It was very bizarre – fascinating – but very bizarre. I didn't know what to think. I felt I knew the baby inside, but who was this? It took a while to get used to her.'

Falling in love with a baby – no matter how desperately wanted – can take time. It can take a few days, it can even take a few weeks. It's entirely understandable that so many first-time mothers feel a little 'freaked out' by this new person, to say the least.

The one piece of advice I will pass on was from one mother who was so 'freaked out' that she forgot to pick the baby up, smile at him and cuddle him. She says, 'When I look at photographs from the day he was born I am horrified. He is next to me but I'm not holding him. I am dressed in a nightie and a dressing gown and he is wearing a sleep suit. I was so blown away by the whole experience I forgot to do skin-to-skin. I didn't even smile at him.'

Even if you are feeling too sore or exhausted to hold the baby, you can lie on your side with him right next to you. This allows you both to nap in very close proximity and enjoy each other's smells and breathing. Another time to focus on this new being is during breastfeeding, when you can study his profile, little ear, arm and body.

So, fear not. You will get the magic moments back. You will get a chance to bond and fall in love with your baby. Being a mother is not straightforward, and this is perhaps your first experience of that important lesson.

your baby's immediate medical care

FIRST CHECKS

Very soon after your baby is born, medical staff will carry out a few checks to establish that your baby is healthy.

APGAR The Apgar score was developed by Dr Virginia Apgar, an American anaesthetist and paediatrician, and is an assessment of the baby's physical condition carried out by a midwife or neonatal doctor one minute after the birth, five minutes after the birth, and again at 10 minutes after the birth. The baby will be scored out of 10 on the following: colour; respiratory rate; muscle tone; reflex irritability; heart rate.

Most babies born at term have scores of nine one minute after the birth, then 10 at the next check. The first score is nine because their hands and feet can take a little while to gain their colour and 'pink up'. An initial score of seven or over indicates that the baby is in good shape. A score of six or less indicates baby has had birth asphyxia (reduced oxygen). If the baby still scores less than seven after five minutes, it may mean the baby needs to be referred for neurological checks.

A score of three or less at one minute after birth indicates the baby needs active full resuscitation. Midwives will always have the necessary equipment to resuscitate. If you are at the hospital, a specialist neonatal doctor will be called to assist.

The scores given to your baby will be written in your birth record.

ALL-OVER CHECK As well as the Apgar score, your baby will have a brief all-over check to ensure everything is in order. The face, eyes, mouth, abdomen, spine and genitals will all be checked. Later your baby will be checked again to see that he or she has passed meconium (the black oily first poo of a newborn) and urine. The baby's cord will also be clamped more securely. Either the same day, the following day or within 72 hours, a full check will be done by a paediatrician (see below).

VITAMIN K

Immediately after the birth, you will be asked if you are happy for your baby to receive Vitamin K, either in the form of an injection, or in an oral dose.

Babies are born with very low levels of Vitamin K and there is very little Vitamin K in breast milk, which makes newborns at risk from Vitamin K deficiency. In rare cases – one in 10,000 – a baby can develop haemorrhagic disease, which causes spontaneous bleeding beneath the baby's skin or elsewhere in the body. This is almost completely preventable. It is recommended that your baby is given Vitamin K by injection at birth, and in this case, she will only need one dose. However, Vitamin K can also be taken orally and, if you take this option and also choose to breastfeed exclusively, your baby will need to be given Vitamin K at birth, again at 7 days, then again at 30 days of life.

NEONATOLOGIST'S CHECK

A neonatologist (paediatrician) will see your baby within 72 hours of the birth. He or she will examine the baby and this will take place in front of you in a warm well-lit area. You may be asked a few questions, such as how you feel about the baby's health, how you felt about your pregnancy and a few general queries about the family's health. The doctor will then tell you about further screening tests, the hearing test, BCG, the vaccination against tuberculosis, and the Guthrie Test (now called Blood Spots).

bathing and cord care

Your midwife will show you how to bath your baby, holding her under the far arm, with her neck resting on your wrist. Keep the water at body temperature (37–37.4°C). Babies do not need to be bathed everyday – in fact it can dry out their skin. However, some mothers like to introduce the bath as part of a nightly routine. You can use a few drops of extra virgin olive oil or pure almond oil in the water. Newborns – particularly those who are overdue – are prone to dry, cracked skin.

Your midwife will also show you how to care for your baby's cord stump before you leave the hospital. Keep the area around the clamp dry and it will fall off naturally within a week.

BCG

The BCG, a vaccination against tuberculosis (TB), is offered routinely in London boroughs where there is a high risk of TB. You can say no to this injection.

HEARING TEST

All babies in the UK now have their hearing checked immediately after birth. The test can be done while the baby is quiet or asleep. The screener will place a small device in the baby's ear that will send sound frequencies into the inner ear. These then produce an echo that the screening equipment will pick up. If you have a 'clear' response, it is unlikely that the baby has hearing problems. If one ear doesn't have a clear response – which can happen even when there is nothing wrong – the test will be repeated.

If the ears are blocked by gunge, you will have to wait until this clears up before repeating the test. You will be given the results and, if any follow-up is necessary, any further contacts you need.

NEONATAL JAUNDICE

Jaundice affects 60% of term babies and 80% of preterm babies to varying degrees. Breastfed babies are more likely to have it, as are boys. The primary symptom of jaundice is a yellowing of the skin and the whites of the eyes – people often comment that the baby looks 'tanned'.

Jaundice is caused when the baby's liver struggles to break down excess red blood cells it no longer needs after birth, and it is treated with sunlight (which is why midwives often tell you to put your baby near the window) or UV light as well as regular feeds.

There are also two types of the condition: physiological or pathological. Pathological, which is the more worrying of the two, occurs within the first 24 hours of birth. If you notice your baby becoming jaundiced within the first 24 hours, seek advice. In very rare cases high levels of jaundice can cause kernicterus, or jaundice of the brain, which in turn causes brain damage.

Physiological jaundice occurs within two to five days and usually goes by 10 days. The baby will let you know if he is unwell – he won't feed well, he won't pass urine, he will be floppy and listless and sleep too much. If you do have any concerns, speak to your midwife, health visitor or GP. Tests can be done to check the levels of bilrubin and work out the cause of the jaundice. In extreme cases, the baby may require phototherapy and exchange blood transfusions.

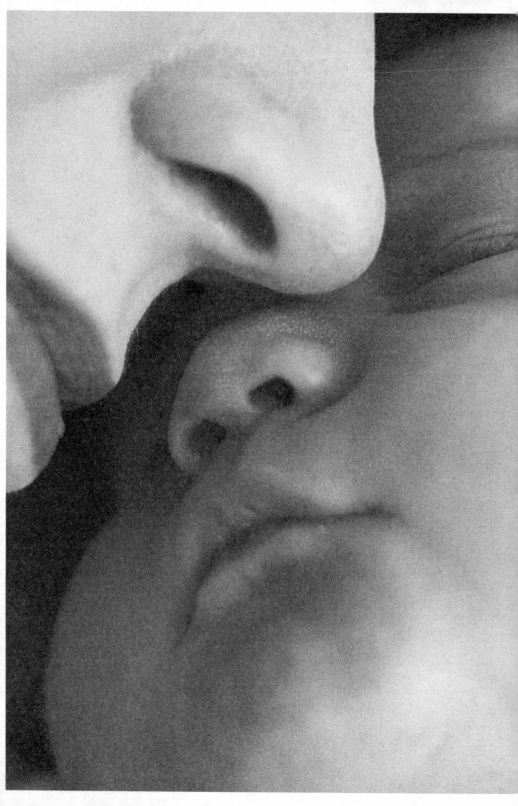

PART THREE

your
baby

the first six weeks

In the coming weeks, exhilaration and exhaustion go hand-in-hand. This is a time for snuggling down at home and getting to know your gorgeous baby more and more as every day passes, and as he changes from a tiny, delicate little newborn cradled in your arms to a six-week-old baby, eager to see your face and to take in the world around him.

your baby is here!

Your baby is a 'newborn' for such a short period – and it goes so fast. Her smell, the curled up hands, squashed face and squinting eyes – these will all go over the next six weeks and she will grow at an extraordinarily rapid pace. It's a time of your life you will never forget, a time of profound change. Cherish it and take your time to get to know your baby. There's no need to rush, just take each day as it comes.

Becoming a parent is both terrifying and empowering. You should feel proud of yourself and of your gorgeous little baby.

LEAVING THE HOSPITAL

You've been through the checks and both you and your baby have been signed off. You've been through the essentials of care with the midwife and you've changed your first (and probably second, third and fourth) nappy. Now the car seat is in the car, the baby is dressed to go outside for the first time and you're about to go home with your new baby. This is the point at which so many new mothers feel suddenly struck with panic.

More than once a mother has said to me, 'Jenny can you come home with me?' My response is, 'Don't worry, you'll be fine.' And of course you will be. Take a few deep breaths and think to yourself 'this is a whole new adventure'.

YOUR ONGOING CARE

Your midwife, or a 'community midwife', will look after you for between 10 and 28 days after the birth. She (and it usually is a she) will be primarily concerned with your recovery, the baby's feeding routine, the baby's weight, jaundice, cord care and any problems you may have with breastfeeding, such as mastitis.

At any point from 10 days onwards, the health visitor, along with the GP, will take over your care. A health visitor is a registered nurse with midwifery experience who may also have a midwifery qualification. He or she will be responsible for the baby's immunizations, monitoring weight gain and regular health checks. The health visitor's other responsibilities are to detect ill health in mothers and babies as well as any deterioration of physical or mental health, report any physical, mental or social concerns to the relevant agency and help families with health education.

SURRENDER TO THE PINK BUBBLE

It may seem that the baby has taken over your whole life. This little being is small enough to sleep in a basket, yet the whole household is revolving around it. You wonder where the 'me' time is – perhaps you feel you can't even find time to have a shower.

For the first six weeks you just need to rest and look after yourself and the baby. Don't worry about 'getting your life back' – it will come, bit by bit. Surrender to what I call 'the pink bubble'. It's all a bit hazy and there's a rose-tint to it, even when you feel you couldn't get more tired. It may not feel like it now but this is a remarkably short amount of time in your life. Gradually you will find yourself remerging from the bubble. Perhaps it will be a lunch with a friend while someone else watches the baby. Perhaps it will be your first dinner out with your partner. Even just a coffee and a gentle stroll around the park can make you feel as if you are reasserting your independence and identity.

CROWD CONTROL

When you have a new baby everyone wants to visit. Suddenly you are an exhausted mum and a hostess, running around making tea, offering cake and biscuits and trying to make polite conversation. This is the very last thing you need right now. Visitors never mean to impose, they may forget your needs in their excitement to see the baby. Parents and parents-in-law may be a little more tricky: sometimes they feel it is their right to see the baby whenever they like.

My advice is to prepare friends and relatives in advance. Explain that you are planning to have time alone together to get to know the baby. If they are going to pop in, ask them to make it brief – perhaps the length of one cup of tea. Stagger the number of visitors you have over a few weeks. If you are lucky enough to have friends who are very helpful and unobtrusive, it's obviously not necessary to prevent them coming over.

You can also:

⊙ leave the answerphone on
⊙ text/email a photo of the baby to everyone and say you'll be in touch soon
⊙ ask guests who are coming to make you a cup of tea and to bring cake or, even better, a meal for you and your partner with them.

breastfeeding

Breastfeeding is wonderful for both you and the baby and I agree with the government recommendation that, where possible, it is best to breastfeed as much as you possibly can for the first six months of the baby's life.

Information on breastfeeding can be confusing. In addition to the advice given to you by midwives, there are leaflets, lactation consultants, books, pamphlets and support groups. It can feel a little overwhelming. For this reason I am going to try to keep my advice as simple as possible. What works for someone else may not work for you, so don't be put off if your first attempt isn't your best.

THE FIRST HOUR

If possible, try to feed as soon as your baby arrives. Keep your baby skin-to-skin and near your breasts to increase the chances of him or her breastfeeding within the first hour. Babies tend to be more alert in this period.

GETTING STARTED The key to success is positioning and attachment. With your baby held to your breast in position, support the breast with thumb on top and four fingers underneath. Stroke the baby's cheek to stimulate the rooting reflex. Now brush your nipple over her mouth. When your baby makes a 'wide mouth' she should grasp the nipple and the areola. You should be able to see her bottom lip curling back while she sucks. The baby's jaw should move up to the ear and the cheek should be rounded. Hug your baby tightly with a straight back so her neck isn't twisted as she feeds. When finished, your nipple should look like a jelly tot, as opposed to a used lipstick. Use cushions to support you.

tips for successful breastfeeding

- ⊙ Feed from birth and frequently.
- ⊙ Breastfeed on demand to begin with, making sure the baby has at least six to eight feeds in 24 hours.
- ⊙ The whole nipple, including the areola, the area around the nipple, needs to be in the baby's mouth.

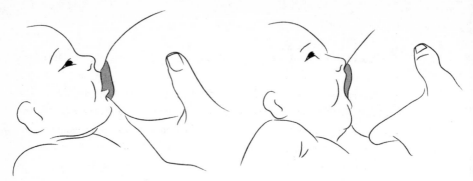

incorrect feeding position   correct feeding position

THE BENEFITS OF BREASTFEEDING

For your baby:

- ☉ Breast milk is specifically made for your baby: it contains the right balance of fat, sugar, protein and water.
- ☉ It contains antibodies that help your baby fight viruses and bacteria. Breastfed babies are better able to fight diarrhoea, ear and chest infections.
- ☉ Breastfed babies are less prone to weight problems later in life.
- ☉ Premature babies who are breastfed do better than premature babies fed on formula
- ☉ Breastmilk is sterile, which helps prevent infections from bottles.

For you:

- ☉ Breastfeeding helps your uterus return to normal more quickly.
- ☉ It is quick and convenient.
- ☉ It helps you lose weight.
- ☉ It lowers your risk of breast cancer.
- ☉ It helps you bond with your baby.

WHEN IS BREASTFEEDING NOT RECOMMENDED?

Do not breastfeed if:

- ☉ you have HIV, because it can be passed to the baby
- ☉ you are addicted to or have taken recreational drugs such as heroin, cocaine or marijuana

- ☉ you are drunk on alcohol
- ☉ you are taking prescribed drugs that are contraindicated for breastfeeding, such as some antibiotics
- ☉ you become ill, such as with a burst appendix, and the milk becomes toxic
- ☉ if your baby has galactosaemia, and cannot break down the galactose in breastmilk. In this situation your paediatrician will recommend a special milk that your baby can digest.

establishing a feeding routine

Feed your baby 'on demand' while you build up your milk supply and get to grips with breastfeeding. Breastfeeding works on a supply and demand basis. In order to maintain your supply, your baby needs to be put on the breast around eight times in a 24-hour period. Most women find that their supply is better in the morning than the evening. Breast milk also flows more readily if the mother is relaxed and calm (so try dimming the lights and some calming breathing exercises if you have any concerns about your milk flow). You also need to eat well to maintain a good supply of milk – approximately 500 extra calories a day – and drink plenty of fluids.

Many women keep a little notebook by the bed writing down the time the baby fed, for how long and from which breast. This can remind you to alternate breasts and help you see if the baby is putting himself into a little routine. In the first few days, you should find that he is feeding three-hourly. If you want to keep him alert so that he completes a feed, one tip is to change his nappy before you switch to the other side.

Once the two of you are practised at breastfeeding, you may want to impose some structure onto that routine so that you are getting the majority of feeds in during the day and the baby is sleeping for longer between feeds at night. Or you may prefer to follow your baby's lead and not impose a feeding routine.

There are endless books on baby routines and, once again, this is yet another politically charged area of babycare – some people argue vehemently for routine, others are equally vociferous against them. You will have to make up your own mind.

My concern as a midwife is to establish whether or not the baby is getting enough milk. This is very hard to judge when you are breastfeeding. By six weeks he will probably be draining both breasts (so that he or she is getting both the thirst-quenching 'foremilk' and the fatty 'hind milk') and not dropping off shortly after the feed has started.

EXPECT THE UNEXPECTED

I think you should breastfeed as much as you can for as long as you can. 'As you can' is a caveat because I don't believe any woman should be held to ransom over the 'breastfeed exclusively' argument. If you are exhausted and the baby has a formula feed – well, it's not the end of the world.

There is a lot of trial and error when it comes to breastfeeding and many women find that, even when they impose a routine, the baby has other ideas. Some babies prefer a particular breast, some a particular position, some will only feed if the environment is completely quiet and relaxed, whereas others wouldn't care or even notice if a war was on when intent on feeding. If you have a baby who feeds all night and you are anxious about imposing a strict routine, you may want to gently push him to do more day feeds so both mother and baby and all can enjoy some wonderful sleep.

Try waking your baby every three hours during the day so that you can stretch out the time between feeds at night. By two months, she should only need to feed once or twice at night.

HOW CAN I BE CERTAIN MY BABY IS GETTING ENOUGH MILK?

Look for the following signs if you need to reassure yourself that your baby is feeding well:

- ⊙ your supply is good
- ⊙ she is gaining weight
- ⊙ her urine is pale yellow (not concentrated)
- ⊙ her poo is mustard yellow
- ⊙ she is alert and interested.

If you are uncertain, talk to your midwife, health visitor or GP and attend regular weigh-ins at the baby clinic.

problems with breastfeeding

SORE NIPPLES

Sore nipples are a common side effect of breastfeeding in the early days and weeks. This can lead to pain when the baby is attaching. Although it is said that breastfeeding should not be uncomfortable if the baby is latched on properly, for some women, myself included, it is uncomfortable for the first 10 seconds. The use of nipple shields remains controversial and they should only be used if you have very sore nipples, as they can reduce milk supply. However, on a very short-term basis they can be useful, allowing your nipples a little rest and respite.

WHAT CAN I DO? I usually tell women to scrunch their toes and breathe deeply as the baby goes on. If the pain subsides after ten or so seconds, you should have a good latch. If not, you may need to reposition the baby.

If you experience bleeding nipples, it may be because the positioning is not perfect and you need to check that the baby has the whole nipple, including the areola, in his mouth (see the diagram on page 294). Don't worry about the baby swallowing some of the blood, or seeing it in his or her 'spit up'. If after a couple of attempts you still have a bad latch, don't panic. Try again. The baby may get agitated but try not to let this frustrate you. Be patient, take a deep breath and try again. If after several attempts, the position you are using isn't working for you, try another. Changing positions helps vary the pressure on different parts of your nipple and also helps the breast drain properly.

You can use breast milk to relieve the pain of stinging nipples or apply topical salves such as Lansinoh, which are specifically for cracked and painful nipples. Avoid using soap on the painful area as it can aggravate it, and wash your bras in non-biological powder.

SORE BREASTS

Before a feed your breasts will feel full, and you may feel a strong urge to feed. Afterwards, they feel 'drained'. An excessive feeling of fullness is known as engorgement and can be very painful. Generally, it first occurs around three to five days after birth. Engorgement is caused by a build up of milk and blood and causes painful, hard breasts.

WHAT CAN I DO? You need to get the milk flowing again and the best way to do this is with very warm water. Either stand under a warm shower and express using your hands or a hand pump, or use hot flannels on your breasts before you express. Once you have drained your breasts, place a cold compress (such as a gel pad or a savoy cabbage leaf that has been chilled in the fridge) inside your bra.

You should also make sure that your maternity bras fit you properly. If possible, it's worth getting your bra fitted by a professional. They may offer this at your local department store.

BLOCKED MILK DUCTS AND INFECTION (MASTITIS)

If you notice a lump in your breast that is not drained by a feed, you may have a blocked duct. When the skin around the duct starts to redden or is painful, it is usually a sign that you have mastitis or an infected duct. Other symptoms include flu-like symptoms and a fever.

WHAT CAN I DO? You need to unblock the duct, which you can do by making the area warm (either in the shower or with a hot flannel on your breast) and then massaging the lump. It's important to continue breastfeeding regularly to help shift the blockage. You can also massage the area as you feed. Try getting the baby to latch on in different positions to see if that helps.

Paracetamol will help with the fever and with the pain, but you also need to rest, sleep and eat well. If the breast stays red for longer than 24 hours, you need to see the midwife or GP. In many cases antibiotics are needed.

THRUSH OF NIPPLES AND BREAST TISSUE

Thrush is a yeast infection (Candida) which thrives on milk. If your nipples crack, the thrush can get into the skin and cause shooting pains when you feed. Women have described wanting to pull the baby from the breast, it's so sore. Symptoms include flaky skin, redness and tiny blisters. Thrush is particularly bad because it can pass into the baby's body, into his or her mouth and bottom, which will then become sore.

WHAT CAN I DO? See your GP as soon as possible and get treatment in the form of creams for your nipples and medicine for the baby. Keep the area meticulously clean and regularly change your clothes – especially your bra – and any towels or flannels that come into contact with the area. Wash your hands as often as possible.

BABY REFUSES TO FEED
Usually, a baby that doesn't want to feed is trying to tell you something. Below is a quick checklist of common problems:

- ⊙ he has a blocked nose
- ⊙ he has an ear infection
- ⊙ he is unwell
- ⊙ he is too hot
- ⊙ the mother is too stressed and 'let down' is not immediate
- ⊙ there is too much surrounding noise
- ⊙ you are chatting (babies are often particularly offended when Mum tries to talk on the phone during a feed)
- ⊙ the milk tastes funny – perhaps you have eaten something with a strong taste that has flavoured your milk.

WHAT CAN I DO?
- ⊙ Give your baby your complete attention.
- ⊙ Check his health – does he seem unwell?
- ⊙ Check his temperature – if necessary remove some of his clothes.
- ⊙ Check his nappy.
- ⊙ Try skin-to-skin contact and dimming the lights.
- ⊙ Get into a warm, candle-lit bath with your baby. It will help you to calm down and prompt the 'let down' reflex. Try different positions and make sure you are both comfortable.
- ⊙ Take pain relief if your nipples are sore.
- ⊙ Express some milk and offer it to your baby in a bottle.
- ⊙ Seek advice from your midwife, health visitor or local representative of La Leche League (see page 328 for contact details).

caring for your newborn

Like all things baby-related, there are probably as many different opinions on how to do things as there are parents. And like all parents, you will find your own way through all the debates and issues. The most important thing is that your baby is safe, well cared for and loved. Below I have run through a general list of baby-care issues.

CARE OF THE UMBILICAL STUMP

After birth, the umbilical cord is cut and a plastic clamp applied close to your baby's abdomen. The plastic clamp can be removed after a few days, or sometimes it is left until the cord drops off. It's best to keep the cord as dry as possible. Fold the nappy away from the clamp and, if you have a boy, ensure his penis points down into the nappy so that he doesn't wee on the cord and keep it moist. If the cord stump gets gungy, clean around it with damp cotton wool followed by dry cotton wool.

Within 10–21 days the stump becomes dry, then falls off like a dried-up twig, leaving a small raw area that will slowly heal and end up being the base of your baby's tummy button. Occasionally, after the stump has fallen off, there is still some lumpy flesh or 'umbilical granuloma', which may require treatment. As the cord stump has no nerves, this is a painless procedure.

If you are worried about infection, contact your midwife or GP. Symptoms include fever, or your baby being generally unwell, the skin around the area becoming red or inflamed and/or pus appearing around the cord stump.

SUPPORT YOUR BABY'S HEAD AND NECK

Newborns have little or no control of their necks at birth, so their neck needs to be supported or cradled at all times to avoid injury. Be careful when you lift your baby out of the cot, and if you put her on your shoulder, be sure to support her with a hand over the neck and back to prevent her from falling backwards. Over time, as the muscles of the neck build up, she will become better at supporting her own head.

Secure car seats properly and make sure you have a neck support fitted. Also make sure that the baby carriers are tight when you are walking so that the neck does not wobble.

THE BABY'S WEIGHT

When your baby is born, everyone wants to know how much he or she weighed. It's almost as if the baby's weight is a defining characteristic – people even put the weight on the birth announcement card. In some ways it is quite bizarre.

The interest in the baby's weight, however, continues over the first 12 weeks and, this time, it is for a very good reason. It is important that your baby is putting on enough weight and that this gain is following the expected trajectory (on a 'centile' chart). Babies often lose around 10% of their birth weight in the first few days after birth, before starting to put it back on at quite a pace. They are usually back to their birth weight within 10 days but your midwife and health visitor will want to regularly check that everything is as it should be.

It's difficult to give a 'one size fits all' weight-gain pattern for all babies, but they should gain roughly 170–225g (6–8oz) a week. In the old days we used to say 'doubling [their birth weight] by six months, tripling by a year'. I think this is still sound advice.

BABY'S POO – IT KEEPS CHANGING COLOUR!

Everything you find in the baby's nappy is directly related to what goes in through his mouth. Initially, your baby only has very small volumes of colostrum, but once your milk comes in, that increases to a more substantial amount, which means more nappies. Babies who are breastfed have different poos to those on formula milk.

DAYS 1–2 Your baby will pass meconium, a black or dark green, odourless, tarry stool, and only very small amounts of urine.

DAYS 3–4 You will notice your baby's poos change to a greenish/yellow colour. He may start to wee up to five times a day.

DAYS 5–7 His poo is watery in consistency and mustardy in colour, often with 'seeds'. This is typical breastfed baby poo and it has a faint 'nutty' odour. It will be what you come to expect from a nappy until he is weaned. He may be weeing five to six times a day.

THINGS TO NOTE:

⊙ If you are suffering from cracked or bleeding nipples, you may notice small

streaks of red in the baby's poo.
- ⊙ If your baby passes very mucousy stools consult your midwife, as this can happen if your baby suffers from cystic fibrosis.
- ⊙ If the poo is very green, your baby may not be getting enough 'hind' milk – the thick protein-rich milk that comes after the thirst-quenching 'foremilk'. Try keeping the baby on each breast for longer to make sure he is getting everything he needs.
- ⊙ If you start breastfeeding and then switch to formula, your baby may not poo for a whole day because of the change in diet.

TO SWADDLE, OR NOT TO SWADDLE?

Babies have been swaddled for centuries in various cultures and the idea behind swaddling is that it recreates the womb-like restrictions and makes the baby feel secure. A recent study on swaddling[20] found that the practice helped babies stay on their backs (the recommended sleeping position for all babies, to reduce the risk of cot death), and that they were more likely to sleep for longer. Researchers concluded that 'Swaddling promotes more sustained sleep and reduces frequency of spontaneous awakenings.'

You can swaddle your baby with a stretchy cotton blanket or, when it is bitterly cold, a cellular blanket. There are many different methods and you need to find the one that you do best. The smaller the baby, the easier it is to swaddle. As your baby gets bigger you may want to introduce the half swaddle (one arm out) and then let her have both arms out before moving her to a baby sleeping bag. Two of my babies preferred having their arms out from the outset, and this can be a good compromise for a baby that isn't entirely convinced by swaddling.

In my opinion it makes perfect sense to swaddle baby until at least eight weeks, but I issue three points of caution.

- ⊙ Not every baby likes to be swaddled. Some babies loathe it and cry or battle even a half-swaddle. In this case, you can introduce the sleeping bag as an alternative. The advantage of sleeping bags over duvets or sheets and blankets is that your baby, particularly if he or she is a wriggler, is not at risk of either becoming tangled in the bedclothes or of overheating. Make sure you use a sleeping bag with the right 'tog' for the season.
- ⊙ Don't let the baby overheat. If your baby is overdressed and then you

swaddle them too, she could get too hot and, as we know, newborns are not good at regulating their own temperature. If you are swaddling with a stretchy cotton cloth, make sure you adapt the clothes the baby is wearing underneath it to the season. If it is the middle of a bitter winter, you can always place a thin cellular blanket over the top of your swaddled baby, and tuck it in tightly on both sides of the mattress so it doesn't accidentally climb over the baby's head.

⊙ Finally, you need to recognize when it's time to stop swaddling her and move her into a sleeping bag. This is usually anytime beyond eight weeks, depending on the baby.

DUMMIES: GOOD OR BAD?

Here is another subject that brings out extreme reactions in some mothers and childcare manuals. As a result, you may already have formed an opinion. In general, it probably is better if dummies are avoided. However, you never know how your baby is going to be and it might be that you finally introduce it as a last resort after many sleepless nights. Other parents have told me, with some frustration, that their second or third child just wouldn't take it, spitting it out each time they tried. So, it may also be that your own view on dummies differs from your baby's.

Some professionals argue that introducing a dummy before the first month can interfere with breastfeeding. I've not personally seen evidence of this. Others argue that, so long as the dummy is taken away by the end of four months, the baby won't be 'addicted'. Again, this may be the case for some babies and not for others.

One study by a senior research scientist in California, suggested that the use of dummies could reduce the risk of Sudden Infant Death Syndrome (SIDS, also called cot death), and could possibly reduce the influence of known risks to the baby, such as smoking parents.[21]

Certainly, once the baby is asleep, the dummy is redundant, so one way of reducing dependence may be to use it only as a way of getting the baby off to sleep, and then spirit it away.

Frequent and prolonged use is not recommended because it can affect the baby's tooth development and speech development (because it stops the baby from babbling as much).

TAKING YOUR BABY OUTSIDE

Your first trip outside is usually the journey home from the hospital. The next time you go out may depend on a number of factors – not least the weather. You need to feel ready yourself, particularly if you had an exhausting birth and you are still sore, but I think a newborn can go out in good weather anytime from day five. It might be an idea to keep the trip local so you can go home if you feel the need.

My cautions are as follows.

- Avoid anyone who is unwell.
- Ask everyone to wash their hands before holding the baby (you can also buy antiseptic hand gel and keep it in your handbag).
- Avoid loud, busy places where the baby may catch an infection.
- Avoid anywhere that is smoky.
- Avoid busy roads.
- Avoid direct sunlight – especially in summer. You can pin a muslin to the pram hood to prevent the baby getting burnt.

entertaining your baby

Babies need communication and age-appropriate stimulation. Here are some suggestions for the first six weeks.

- Look into your baby's eyes, holding him about 8in away from you.
- Make faces at him – raising eyebrows, sticking out your tongue, smiling.
- Massage him with olive oil, gently stroking arms, legs, feet and hands.
- Dance with your baby, swirling and rocking in gentle, smooth movements.

- Play music.
- Place mobiles or patterned pictures about 8in away from his face.
- Introduce him to different-textured fabrics – silky, crunchy – and give him a variety of age-appropriate toys to explore.
- Rock him in a pram.
- Have a bath with him.
- Take him for a walk in the part and talk to him about what he can see and hear – different trees, changes in the sky, children playing, birds twittering.

DRESSING THE BABY

Both over- and under-dressing the baby pose risks. While grandparents may think babies are under-dressed, the reason we do not over-wrap them is that they cannot regulate their own temperature. Babies don't sweat to bring their temperature down, and don't shiver to bring it up, so they are entirely dependent on us to keep them comfortable. The best way to test whether your baby is too hot or too cold is by checking his or her 'core temperature' on the chest or back. If this area is warm then they are fine, if it is hot, they are not. If your baby feels very hot, strip off their clothes until their temperature returns to normal. I usually say that the baby needs one more layer than you do.

It's very important that your baby doesn't get cold all over as this can cause hypothermia. Check both their extremities and their core temperature to determine if they are cold – they may have coldish feet and hands but a very warm body, in which case they need socks and booties as opposed to another blanket or layer of clothing.

CIRCUMCISION

Circumcision of male babies is not done routinely in the UK as it is in the United States, where between 50–60% of male babies are circumcised at birth. In the UK it is thought that around 15% of male babies are circumcised, the vast majority of those will be Jews and Muslims who circumcise for religious reasons.

The debates around circumcision for non-religious reasons are constantly changing. Female circumcision is banned in the UK under the 1985 Prohibition of Female Circumcision Act.

BABY MASSAGE

Baby massage has a wealth of benefits for both mother and baby and is a wonderful way to bond and help the baby relax. It's also thought to improve colic and aid sleep in babies.

Baby massage is taught throughout the UK. Contact your local branch of the National Childbirth Trust for details (see page 328 for contact details).

your post-partum health

Well done! Your body is amazing. You have nurtured this baby from the tiny beginnings of life into the bundle of joy that is now in your arms. So, even if things didn't go completely to plan and you feel rather worse for wear on the other side, congratulate yourself on this incredible achievement.

Your body probably doesn't feel much like your own at this point – it's been through some of the most dramatic changes to date. Now you will be experiencing a drop in the pregnancy hormones and, if you are breastfeeding, a blast of the 'love hormones' mixed with exhaustion, and some fears about being able to cope.

It's all part of the journey. Below I have listed some of the common complaints and made suggestions on how to deal with your body in new motherhood.

YOUR BREASTS

For the first two to three days after birth, you will be producing colostrum, a yellowy-white pre-milk breast milk that is very high in antibodies and helps your baby's immune system. Oestrogen levels fall, corresponding with a rise in prolactin (the hormone that allows milk production). Women often say they woke on the third day with breasts as hard as wood – this is when your milk has 'come in'.

Your breasts – which may have already grown a few sizes during pregnancy – will now feel very full with blood and milk and, if you haven't already, you will need to invest in a nursing bra. If you find you leak milk you may also need breast pads, which are available at the chemist.

YOUR STITCHES

Stitches after childbirth are extremely common. In some cases, they are relatively painless, but many women find the area is sore, swollen and tender for a few days. Stitches take about three weeks to dissolve, but even those who did not have stitches may be feeling discomfort. Below are some tips.

⊙ **Keep the area clean and dry to prevent infection. Loose clothing is better so that the perineal area doesn't get sweaty, which would keep the stitches** moist. Change your maternity pad regularly and wear cotton knickers when the bleeding subsides.

- Eat a good diet – this aids tissue repair.
- When passing urine, you may feel a stinging sensation. Try squirting water onto the area from a plastic bottle with a sports cap.
- For the first week after birth you may feel an unpleasant 'pulling' sensation as you take each step up or down the stairs. While it is good to move around (it keeps your circulation going and prevents blood clots) try, as much as possible, to avoid stairs for the first few days.
- Avoid standing too long as fluid can build up in the area and make the swelling worse.
- Keep up those pelvic floor exercises – they boost circulation.
- Take natural pain relief – arnica tablets help reduce swelling and bruising and drops of lavender oil or tea tree oil in the bath can be very soothing.
- If the pain is bad, you can take paracetamol, co-dyromol (although these can cause constipation) or voltoral tablets or suppositories (although the latter are contraindicated if you are asthmatic or have had stomach ulcers).

BLEEDING (LOCHIA)

In the first few days after birth the bleeding is pronounced and some midwives recommend a double maternity towel. At this stage it is usually fresh red blood and dead cells from the uterine lining, but this is replaced by a pinkish blood and then brown (old) blood over the course of the next week or so.

Most women continue to experience small amounts of brownish blood loss for two weeks after that. Some women – particularly those who have had previous babies or a Caesarean section – may continue to get red or pink blood again for up to six weeks post partum. Other women also experience a whitish discharge for up to a month after the birth. That is all normal.

I have a few notes of caution.

- If you pass small or large clots or membrane, tell your midwife. She will want to rule out any risk of placental tissue being left in your womb. If there are so-called 'retained products', you may need to be scanned and given a course of antibiotics.
- If you are getting strong red bleeding again over a week after the birth, this can be a sign that you are doing too much. Take it easy.

- If the bleeding is accompanied by a bad or unusual 'fusty' smell, tell your midwife immediately. This is usually a sign of an infection.
- Do not use tampons for the first six weeks after birth because they can cause bacteria to build up and cause infections.
- Be careful to keep your iron levels up – you don't want to risk becoming anaemic. A good iron supplement may work for you.

THE CAESAREAN SCAR

A Caesarean is still a big operation and you need to recover. You will probably stay in hospital for anything from two to five days and you will need to take regular pain relief as your wound heals.

Most Caesareans are carried out with an epidural so you can have doses of epidural top up immediately afterwards. After two hours in a recovery room, your wound will be checked as will your maternity pads and, all being well, you will then be transferred to the postnatal ward or your room.

Dressings are not usually removed for two days and my advice is to shower first and let the dressing get wet so that it is less sore when it's removed. In most cases, your wound will require no further attention until day five, when the subcuticular suture is removed.

It takes up to six weeks for the wound to properly heal and it may look red for some time before fading to a silvery line, not unlike a stretch mark.

Keep an eye out for the following signs of problems.

- If you feel unwell during the recovery time or if you are losing a lot of blood, make sure you tell the midwives or doctor. This is not a good sign.
- If the wound bleeds a lot or if it gets red, sore and inflamed, you may have an infection developing and you need to seek medical help and get antibiotics.
- If your wound is 'gaping' – this may mean you need surgical packs or re-suturing. See your doctor as soon as you can.

BREASTFEEDING AFTER A CAESAREAN It is easier to lie on your side to feed the baby, so that the baby's weight is not on your abdomen. Other methods are to feed holding the baby under arm, in what is called the 'rugby hold' (this is also used for twins).

LIFTING It's very important not to strain your tummy muscles in the first six weeks, so please don't carry older children (you can sit down and they can climb up for a hug), heavy shopping and don't move any furniture – including the Moses basket. The hormone progesterone can still cause stretching of the ligaments and you can be at risk of serious backache and sciatica.

DRIVING Don't drive for the first six weeks, because your wound is at risk each time you use the brake. Your reflexes and reactions may be slowed by the pain, which makes driving dangerous. It's worth noting that your insurance company will not pay for any damage you do to the car if you drive in the first six weeks after a Caesarean section.

HAEMORRHOIDS

Haemorrhoids, or piles, can occur during childbirth because of the pushing. They can also happen afterwards. Shortly after the birth you may find it difficult to do a poo, and the first bowel movement is often difficult and painful. Most women fear 'everything will fall out', particularly if they are sore and swollen. Others 'can't go'. I usually tell them to hold a sanitary pad against the front of their perineum for support – the help is more psychological than physical, but it really does work.

You can get immediate relief from ice or gel packs, or just a bag of frozen peas, but you will probably want to get a topical cream from the chemist in order to treat the haemorrhoids properly. Lignocaine gel can numb the area if you are in great pain. You can use a special rubber ring to sit on, but I recommend that you use it only for 30 minutes at a time as it can restrict circulation around your bottom, making the swelling and long-term discomfort worse. And don't forget your pelvic floor exercises. (See also pages 37–8.)

AFTERPAINS

Once you have delivered the placenta, your uterus, which was below your rib cage, drops to roughly the level of your tummy button. You can touch it if you press into your tummy – it feels round and hard like a cricket ball.

Over the next 10–14 days, your uterus will contract back to its former pre-pregnancy size in a process called 'involution'. You will actually feel this happening – and it feels stronger and more painful with each subsequent pregnancy – particularly when you are breastfeeding. This is because the action that allows the uterus to squeeze down in size is helped by oxytocin, which is released during breastfeeding.

If your afterpains feel excruciating, seem to be going on for longer than a week, or if you feel any tenderness at the top of the uterus, seek medical advice. It could be that you have an infection, or that some of the placenta has been retained. In this case, your lochia will also smell offensive.

Your uterus and cervix will always remain slightly larger than they were before you were pregnant.

ADRENALINE FOLLOWED BY TIREDNESS

Adrenaline helps you through the first few days post-birth, but can then tail off. This is why it is so important to rest and not behave like superwoman. Yes, you have achieved something amazing. Yes, you have finally met your baby. And yes, you will be looking radiant. But you do still need to take it easy and look after yourself.

I know many women, particularly those who had an easy birth, who try to do everything immediately afterwards. They get up in the morning, do the shopping, play hostess to all the guests, even look after the other kids. In my view this is a recipe for disaster. You will exhaust yourself after a week and you will find it very difficult to claw back this time later when the cycle of sleep deprivation really kicks in.

REST. And then rest some more. Eat well, relax, listen to nice music, watch television. You need to conserve pockets of energy to draw on in later weeks. You are not supposed to be up and bouncing up and down, you are supposed to be resting and looking after the baby. Your partner needs to be looking after you. Keep visitors to a minimum. Make sure you have a good team of help and support in place – recruit family, friends and even neighbours to help.

Once the cycle of tiredness starts you will really appreciate having paced yourself. When women say that they don't even have time to have a shower and wash their hair after the baby's birth, they are not joking. If you are breastfeeding, you will probably find each feed takes up one whole hour out of every four as baby gets practised.

THE DAY-THREE BLUES

The day-three blues is an entirely hormonal phenonmenon and does not indicate any increase in likelihood that you will suffer from postnatal depression.

I would go as far as to say that it is a normal part of having a baby – although not everyone gets it. The day-three blues coincide with a drop off in the pregnancy hormones oestrogen and progesterone, and a tailing off of the adrenaline that you may have felt around the birth experience. Some women actually describe it as feeling like a 'crash'. The blues are exacerbated by the exhaustion you may be feeling post birth and with interrupted night-time sleep.

There is an element of madness that goes with the post-birth period, so you may feel that these blues have been set off by something relatively trivial – in my case it was that the cap on the toothpaste hadn't been replaced. Things can certainly get out of perspective on very little sleep.

You need maximum support post-birth, so make sure partners, parents and loved ones are around for you at this time. You also need to rest, rest, rest. If you let yourself get too behind on sleep it is very difficult to catch up in the period after birth.

Once again I have a note of caution. If the weepiness continues beyond a few days and you feel as if the bond with the baby is being interrupted, discuss this with your midwife or GP as soon as possible so that they can rule out postnatal depression.

NIGHT SWEATS

It's not just the baby that can wake you up. In the first few days after birth, you may wake up drenched in sweat, your clothes and bed sheets sodden. You may feel very hot, you may also feel cold as a result of the damp.

This is one of the side effects of giving birth and it is caused by hormonal changes, particularly in women who are breastfeeding. The night sweats coincide with an increase in prolactin levels, which produce breast milk, increase your temperature and make you perspire.

It's nothing to be worried about and the only real way to deal with night sweats is by wearing cotton nightclothes and maternity bras and sleeping with as few bedclothes as you can get away with. If you find you are sweating profusely, you could also use a mattress protector – you may already have one if you were worried about your waters breaking before the birth.

Make sure you drink plenty of water during the day and keep a jug by your bed at night, as a combination of breastfeeding and night sweats can leave you dehydrated and with a desert thirst.

I have a few notes of caution:

⊙ Sweating profusely can also be a sign of an infection, such as mastitis (see page 298). Check your temperature to see if it is above 38°C. If it is, you may have an infection and you need to tell your midwife or GP as soon as possible. Infections can occur in the uterus, breasts, bladder or perineum.

⊙ If you are experiencing a prolonged period of night sweating, panic attacks, weepiness, an increased heart rate, or if the night sweats are occurring later than a few days after the birth, you need to see your GP or midwife, because it could be that you are experiencing one of the symptoms of postnatal depression (see opposite).

'BABY WEIGHT' AND THE WOBBLY TUMMY NO ONE WARNED YOU ABOUT

I don't want to dwell for too long on 'baby weight' because I think the fixation with women and their figures immediately post-birth is ridiculous. The majority of women go through exactly the same experience post-birth: you look down at your tummy and, despite the fact the baby has gone, you still look about 20 weeks pregnant. While our bodies are undoubtedly amazing, we still have to give them a little time to fully recover. You will notice that you will lose huge volumes of fluid in the next few weeks and this is part of the recovery process.

The excess skin and fat will recede over a period of weeks, and while some women snap back to their pre-baby shape quite quickly, it takes most women, myself included, around a year.

As with the pregnancy figure, all women are different. Some women lose too much weight while breastfeeding. For others, it is not until they give up that their body returns to normal.

You can start exercising again after your six-week check with the GP. It's important not to do too much of anything before this as it can exacerbate uterine bleeding. Your ligaments are still soft from pregnancy and you can strain yourself quite easily. I recommend keeping up the gentle practices of pregnancy: gentle swimming, yoga and walking.

My personal view is that you should not try to diet straight after the birth; you need every ounce of energy for looking after the baby. If you are breastfeeding, you will need to eat more excess calories than when you were pregnant – around 500 extra a day.

postnatal depression

One mother in ten will suffer from postnatal depression. The incidence peaks at between four and six months after the birth, but it can happen at any time or develop gradually over time. The severity of postnatal depression can also vary. Some women experience it relatively mildly, some find it debilitating and, tragically, some mothers take their own lives.

There is no telling who will get postnatal depression, but it can be triggered by any number of issues, including, the changing role that motherhood brings, the changing relationship with a partner after the birth of the baby, lack of support or of rest, loneliness, a difficult labour or flash backs to childhood experiences.

Among the recognized signs are tiredness, feelings of inadequacy or not being able to cope, irritability, weepiness, difficulty sleeping, loss of appetite, indifference to offers of help from a partner or relatives and disinterest in intimacy or sex. More serious sufferers might also experience panic attacks, loss of concentration, obsessive fears about the baby, an inability to care well for oneself or the baby, or long periods of staring into space.

Health visitors assess all the women in their care using a questionnaire called the Edinburgh Postnatal Depression Scale. This covers a broad range of questions about how you are feeling and rates your risk. It can be very useful and prompt health visitors into referring you for help where necessary.

This is a difficult subject, but the most obvious, and important, thing to say is take good care of yourself. Don't try to be perfect. Don't try to be supermum. If you suspect you may be a sufferer, get help as soon as you can. If you think you may be teetering on the brink of PND, get out of the house and meet other mothers. Seek help from friends or a professional.

If you are a partner reading this, I have some advice for you, too. Don't tell her to pull herself together, get angry with her, threaten to walk out (and definitely don't walk out) or allow her to turn to alcohol. DO get positive help from a professional.

See page 327 for a list of helpful organizations that can offer support.

WHAT HAS HAPPENED TO MY INTIMATE BITS?

This has to be something that crosses every mother's mind at some point shortly after birth. Women worry hugely about what they will look like 'down there' and often anxiously ask whether it's 'all falling open'. When I look, it's actually healing wonderfully.

There may be grazes, cuts both inside and out, and the whole area may be swollen. Initially, torn labia can appear a little lopsided but it doesn't affect function and they do return to something approaching normal. The entrance of the vagina takes a little longer to return to normal, but it does.

Like the excess weight around your tummy, it all gradually calms down. Some women find having a quick look with a mirror immensely helpful because it never looks as bad as you think. Others don't look; they prefer to be cheerily positive.

SEX

Another common question is: will sex ever be the same again? The short answer is: yes. It's generally recommended that you allow a bit of time for your stitches to heal (perhaps three weeks) and for the bleeding to stop, but I do know some women who try sex before that. If you suffered quite bad tearing you will probably want to wait a bit longer.

The first attempt may hurt a little and I recommend everyone, especially those who are breastfeeding, use plenty of lubricant and take it very slowly. After the first few attempts you will feel everything returning to normal – and if it still feels painful, don't be afraid to go to the GP. It could be that you need specialist help, an operation or that your stitches were sewn up too tightly.

In general, women tell me that they feel more confident about their bodies as a result of birth. Studies have shown that although 50% of couples find the frequency of sex halves after a baby, 20% of women say they enjoyed the experience more than they did before they got pregnant[22].

One important caution: I must stress how important it is to use contraception – even if you are breastfeeding. I know it is less likely that you will conceive if you are breastfeeding, but believe me, it happens. Women can be bizarrely fertile after pregnancy.

your baby's day

Your baby will need feeding, warmth, sleep, comfort, love and communication. how the recipe is put together forms the tapestry of life. Individual babies, mothers, fathers, families, siblings and communities will influence the way we bring up our babies.

your baby's sleep

Babies sleep A LOT during the first few weeks. You might find that he is awake for stretches that are longer than you would like at night-time, but that will all settle down at some point over the coming weeks.

sleeping on the back

Babies should always be put to sleep on their backs to reduce the risk of Sudden Infant Death Syndrome. The government's Back To Sleep campaign is thought to have saved the lives of thousands of babies and greatly reduced the incidence of SIDS.

However, one side effect of putting babies on their back all the time is that the back of the head can flatten (plagiocephaly). Swedish researchers came up with the goi goi pillow, which you can get if you are worried about the back of your baby's head flattening (see page 329 for sources).

SUDDEN INFANT DEATH SYNDROME (SIDS)

SIDS, which is widely referred to as 'cot death', is the sudden and unexplained death of a baby aged less than one year. Even with a full investigation, no cause of death can be found. Approximately 500 babies between one and four months old die in the UK each year according to the Foundation for the Study of Infant Deaths (FSID). While we still don't know why so many babies die, there is evidence to show that causes include: the baby stopping breathing suddenly; the abnormal beating of the heart; problems with the medulla in the brain; allergies; toxins; genetic abnormalities. While any baby can be affected, there is an increased risk for premature babies, boys and babies with low birth weights.

The measures you can take to reduce the risk of SIDS are as follows:

- ⊙ don't smoke in pregnancy
- ⊙ don't smoke around the baby or expose him to a smoky environment
- ⊙ if the baby is ill, seek urgent medical help
- ⊙ if the baby is floppy and sleeps too much, get medical help immediately
- ⊙ put the baby to sleep in a cot in your bedroom for the first six months
- ⊙ place the baby on his back to sleep
- ⊙ place the baby's feet near the bottom of the cot
- ⊙ never fall asleep with your baby on the sofa
- ⊙ don't let the baby sleep with a pillow or a duvet
- ⊙ don't let the baby get too hot
- ⊙ take the baby's outdoor clothes off as soon as you get indoors
- ⊙ don't use a hot water bottle
- ⊙ don't share a bed with the baby
- ⊙ keep the room at a temperature of between 18–20°C
- ⊙ one study suggests the use of a dummy may lessen the risk of SIDS.

establishing a routine

Here is yet another baby-care minefield: the politics of the routine. There are shelves of books on sale waiting to lecture you on which routine is the best. Doctors, midwives, maternity nurses and parents all have a version they want you to follow. Of course, the routines stretch from one extreme to the other.

baby clinics

These were first established in the early part of the 20th century and since then they haven't changed much. You can drop in to the clinic on any day during opening hours and have your baby checked and weighed. GPs and health visitors at the clinic can answer a whole range of questions on the baby's health and wellbeing. This is the place for advice on any concerns you have about immunization, feeding, sleeping and general developmental progress.

One maternity nurse may recommend you put the baby in their own room early on, while an eminent obstetrician may encourage you to co-sleep with your child and cite the millions of children around the planet who do the same.

Like those dispensing the advice, each mother is different and will find what suits her. Some women swear by a routine, introducing a feeding schedule from as early as a week or two and putting the baby to bed in their own room. If this sounds like you, you may prefer the ideas in Gina Ford's *The New Contented Little Baby Book* or Tracy Hogg's book *The Baby Whisperer*. The advantage of these approaches is that you have some structure imposed on your day. The first feed is at 7am, the last at 10 or 11pm. It allows your partner to be involved and the goal is to have a baby that sleeps from 7pm to 7am by four months.

Others are vehemently critical of this type of approach, and routines like this are often thought of as strict, rigid and even impossible to follow. These critics include some midwives and health visitors.

At the other end of the spectrum are those that subscribe to the 'attachment parenting' school of thought (recommended by the paediatrician William Sears in his books, for example). This school advocates feeding on demand (even if that means around the clock) and 'co-sleeping' (sharing a bed) with your children. The advantages of this approach is that you may feel that you are as close to your children as you can possibly be – sleeping next to them, watching them breathe, taking in their delicious clean and innocent smell, is just wonderful.

You need to find what works for you. I know mothers who have used one method for one child and swung the other way for the second. You could take a bit from here and a bit from there. In my case I muddled along in my own way. It wasn't necessarily 'right' but it worked for my family and, broadly, I'm happy with how we did things.

co-sleeping

Sleeping separately from babies and children is so ingrained in our culture that it is difficult even to talk about the positive long-term effects of co-sleeping without being laughed at. Government guidelines suggest babies should not sleep in the parental bed to prevent cot death. However, there are many families who, with due caution, have slept with their babies successfully. Parents need to decide what is the best thing to do for their own babies. For myself, as a working mother, I achieved much closeness with my children by sleeping with them at night. If you do choose to sleep with your baby, keep pillows and duvets away from her face.

why babies cry

Babies cry. It is the only way they can let you know something is wrong. Unfortunately, some babies cry more than others, and this can take its toll on a distressed and tired mother who is trying to meet her baby's needs. When your baby cries, try to go through the checklist of things that might be wrong. Consider the following points to see if you can get to the bottom of why your baby is crying and which of his or her needs you can fill.

HUNGER

Is the baby hungry? You may be thinking – but I've already fed her, how can she still be hungry? The answer is that babies go through growth spurts and, for a few days, seem to want to feed more often. Try feeding her and settling her again.

DIRTY NAPPY

A dirty nappy can make some babies very fussy.

NAPPY RASH

Check for redness on the bottom and use a barrier cream if necessary. If it is very sore, it could be a sign of thrush, so see your midwife or GP.

TOO HOT OR TOO COLD?

The room temperature should be between 18–20°C. If it is summer, the baby only needs one layer. If it's cold, the baby needs one more layer than you.

NOT WELL?

Check the baby's temperature, although sometimes a baby can be unwell and have no fever (and vice versa – have a fever and not be very unwell). If you think your baby is very unwell, contact your midwife or GP.

TIRED?

Tiredness is a very common problem. The baby cries because she is tired, so the mother picks her up to soothe her, inadvertently keeping her awake and making her more tired. Dim the lights and get rid of all other stimulation (such as the television, radio, people talking). Preferably move to a room where you are alone with the baby. Shush the baby gently, but don't make eye contact and try to gently bounce or rock her to sleep. Sometimes a gentle rhythmical patting on the bottom can help too, as it reminds them of the beat of your heart in the womb, while the shushing recreates the noise of the blood flowing through the umbilical cord.

IS IT WIND?

Wind can cause tummy ache and crying can actually exacerbate the situation by bringing more air into the tummy. If your baby is pulling his or her legs up or looks slightly off colour around the lips, they may even have colic. There are several ways to wind a colicky baby:

- ☉ try putting the baby over your shoulder and firmly stroking his or her back in an upward motion
- ☉ try patting her back (but don't thump it)
- ☉ walk up stairs with the baby – sometimes it helps wind come up
- ☉ try the Tiger In A Tree position: place the baby's tummy over the inside of your forearm, with the head facing your elbow and your hand holding him or her between the legs. In this position you can stoke baby's back and create a rocking motion with your body. This often relaxes a baby with a sore tummy and is very good for colicky babies
- ☉ sit the baby on your knee and, firmly holding her tummy with one hand and supporting her back and neck with the other, fold them gently forward until they are nearly bent double, and then backwards. Slowly repeat a few times
- ☉ some mothers find going up on tiptoes while simultaneously trying to wind a baby over the shoulder can help
- ☉ try skin-to-skin contact with your baby's tummy against your tummy and bounce gently. The skin-to-skin soothes your baby, while your tummy can help bring up wind
- ☉ apply circular massage on your baby's tummy (although not too hard).

If your baby is regularly crying for long periods of time, ask your partner or a friend to help you out with 'shifts'. If no one else is around and you need to escape the noise for a short amount of time, put the baby in a safe place and close the door. Take deep breaths and try to calm yourself down. Remember the practice we did for labour: bring your shoulders down, breathe deeply, soften your jaw and repeat some of the mantras I recommended for birth – 'everything is going to be fine', 'patience, patience'. If the crying is very bad, try visualisation before going back in. These tactics will make you feel stronger and calmer, and may even help calm the baby. Try also skin-to-skin, try a lullaby and try getting the baby to suck your (clean) finger. If you have a rocking chair you can also sit on that and rock with the baby.

Remember: this time is short in the greater scheme of things, and, in the same way as it's difficult to recall the symptoms of the first trimester, you will soon be out of this time and on to a new chapter of the baby's life. If you are having difficulty coping with regular long bouts of crying, contact the Cry-sis helpline (see page 328 for details).

If you are concerned that there may be something wrong with your baby – and it's okay to trust your instincts – you need to speak to your midwife, GP or health visitor. Your GP can refer you to a paediatrician if necessary.

Some women find cranial osteopathy is a huge help for babies who cry a lot – particularly after a difficult birth. If the baby has spent a long time in the birth canal, it may even be suffering from headaches, which can be treated by a cranial osteopath. Ask your GP to refer you.

becoming a parent

When you're pregnant everyone fusses over you. After you give birth, everyone fusses over the baby. It's a common complaint. However, now that you are a mother you will find yourself increasingly putting your own needs at the back of the queue.

managing your new role as a mother

Some mothers, even grandmothers, are wondering what the real answer is to this question. No textbook has one answer. As I've said so often before, the key to good parenting is patience. A baby cannot help crying, it is still the only way it knows how to vocalize a problem. You will have to wait a good four years – perhaps longer – before you will be able to reason with your child.

Another important attribute is confidence. Think positively – you are an amazing mother and you have just gone through one of life's biggest achievements. Right now you are probably going through some of the best and worst of what motherhood has to offer. Take one day at a time and try not to expect too much of yourself all at once.

In the early days, you may find it takes both parents a long time just to change a nappy, bathe the baby and to negotiate a babygro. In a few weeks' time, you'll be so practised you could do it standing on your head. Some parents like to share all the duties in the early days and do everything together – after all, it's a very romantic time. Later on, it's common for parents to do 'shifts' so that one can rest while the other takes over.

As time goes on, you will find your own way through the onslaught of advice from every direction (even here!). The baby needs to be warm, fed, changed, kept safe, washed and loved – beyond that the decisions are yours to make. You must do what you believe is best for your little family and not worry too much about what others think. We all bring up children differently.

SOME EARLY CHALLENGES
DEAD OF NIGHT ANXIETY It's an odd side effect of birth, but one that women often mention when talking about the first few days with their newborn.

You may find yourself waking up a few times and leaning over the Moses basket to check your baby's breathing. You may suddenly wake up in a panic, wondering if the baby is lost in your bed – you may even find yourself looking in the covers, when actually he or she is sleeping soundly in the cot or Moses basket. Another common fear is that someone has broken into the house.

This is partly because of hormones, and breastfeeding mothers are especially prone to heightened anxiety about the baby's safety. However, as it also happens to fathers, I think it is part and parcel of becoming a parent. Try to reassure yourself: it's normal to worry about the baby's health. This is a sudden and enormous responsibility and everything feels very new. Check the baby if you are worried, but don't let paranoia take over. Sleep is vital at this time – for your own sake and for the sake of the baby. If this problem starts to get out of hand, see the GP.

SCATTINESS A week or so after the birth (as night and day really are blending into one another) you will probably find that the onslaught of the baby's routine has taken over your life. If you are breastfeeding, you may be feeling the effects of what many new mums call 'nappy brain'. This is partially caused by lack of sleep, but is also a side effect of the 'love hormones', which make thinking clearly more of an ambition than a reality for new mums. You'll find it hard to remember appointments, birthdays and to call people back. Washing clothes, bathing, getting the shopping done, even registering the baby's name may all feel unachievable. This is the time when you are most likely to fill up a diesel car with petrol, go to the shop for milk and come back with apples or put the telephone in the fridge.

Most women find that they can manage perhaps one non-baby-related thing per day once the baby arrives. This is where you need to enlist help for the basics such as shopping, cooking and washing.

Two weeks in and you will probably not be able to name the day of the week. This is, of course, completely normal. After six weeks, just as things feel impossible, your baby will start communicating with you – cooing, smiling and even laughing. Things will start to turn a corner as he gets better at feeding and sleeps longer at night. Eight weeks in and you'll feel another landmark has been reached. Things will get easier again at about 12 weeks.

life after birth

Many of the techniques for mentally keeping on top of pregnancy and birth that I discussed previously are equally applicable for life after birth. Of particular importance are relaxation techniques, mantras and breathing exercises.

I've dwelt a lot on looking after yourself physically, but emotional care is also very important at this stretching time of life. If you take care of yourself both emotionally and physically, you'll be better able to take care of your baby, both emotionally and physically. If you've used my advice then by now, my techniques will be second nature to you. However, below I have briefly run through some ideas that may help you now. Use the ideas I have introduced you to – skin-to-skin contact, rituals, snuggly bits, visualisation – to keep your state of mind healthy and positive.

tips for new dads

This section is addressed to Dads who want to support their partners and take an active role in this first part of the baby's life. It is often said that you look after your partner so she can look after the baby. Here's how you can help. Your partner will greatly appreciate it, and you will be doing your baby a service by giving his or her mum a chance to refresh her mind and body. Try any of the following ideas:

- ☉ take over the late evening feed: if your baby is in a routine, perhaps you can do the last feed of the day with expressed milk, while she get an early night
- ☉ change nappies: when the baby is up at night, perhaps you can change the nappy before she feeds the baby
- ☉ give your baby a bath: this is a perfect opportunity for you to have fun and bond with the baby while your partner has a rest
- ☉ sterilize bottles and expressing equipment
- ☉ do the shopping: while she is stuck at home, perhaps you can be in charge of household chores, such as getting food
- ☉ control the guests! You can definitely take charge when it comes to

controlling the number of visitors you have (see Crowd Control, page 292)
- ⊙ control the unwanted advice! You can act as a buffer or interrupt to change a conversation if your partner is getting too many unwanted lectures
- ⊙ look after the baby while your partner gets some well earned 'me' time. This is perhaps the most important help you can give her. Encourange her to pamper herself – go for a manicure with a friend or on a shopping trip to buy something for her post-pregnancy figure. Even a chance to let off steam with a friend is invaluable at this time.

we're parents!

While it may well have been you that gave birth, you both became parents together – and you both have a steep learning curve ahead. It's important to laugh about the strains and stresses and not to take the exhaustion and relentlessness of the situation out on each other. You need each other and you both need to be supportive. Birth throws up many challenges for a Dad too, even if they are different from your own. He may not be used to seeing his wife in a dressing gown all day. He may make silly comments that you will just have to brush off and ignore. He may panic about the responsibilities of fatherhood. These are all things you can get through together.

The baby will get to know Dad, and this is an important role. She will be able to feel how his smell and touch differs from your own. She will learn to feel secure and loved by both parents, despite the subtle differences in approach. As she grows up she may want and need you for different things – if she is ill, she may need mummy. If she wants to run about and be noisy, daddy might be the better option.

... BUT STILL A COUPLE

As well as being parents, you are also still a couple. Find time to have dinner out alone in the first six weeks. Perhaps mum can babysit, perhaps a friend or nanny.

growing together as a family

HOW DO I COPE WITH A BABY AND TODDLER?

If you have an existing child or children, this is the time to enlist help, even the barest minimum. As a mother of four, my advice is to make your life as simple as possible and do what you have to do and no more. The most important things are your health and the happiness of your children. A messy house is merely cosmetic and can be sorted out later.

Don't be afraid of asking those around you – friends, family and neighbours – for help. Perhaps they can cook your supper, take the toddler to the park, take the dog for a walk, do your shopping for you. I know many women feel shy of asking for anything, but this is one time in your life when you have to put your embarrassment to one side.

HOW DO I HELP MY TODDLER COPE WITH THE NEW ARRIVAL?

There are a few tried-and-trusted methods for making your other children feel comfortable with the new arrival.

- When the other children first meet the baby, make sure the baby is not in your arms so that you can greet them with a hug and make a fuss over them and they won't feel as if they have been replaced.
- Encourage the other children to think of a present to buy the baby, and buy them something 'from the baby' too.
- Ask visitors who come to see the baby to make a fuss of the older child before cooing over the baby.
- If they are old enough, involve the other children in the baby's day-to-day routine. Ask them to help by bringing a nappy, cream or muslin – perhaps give a toddler a role, such as 'being in charge' of an aspect of the baby's care. Talk them through what the baby needs and let them ask questions if they are interested.
- If they are not interested, make time to hear what their concerns are. One-to-one time with an older sibling is crucial at this stage in their life.
- While obviously protecting the baby, try not to appear too anxious about the toddler's behaviour around the baby!

references

1 Samuel M Flaxman and Paul W Sherman, *Morning Sickness: A Mechanism for Protecting Mother and Embryo, The Quarterly Review of Biology* (Vol. 75, No.2, pp 113–148, June 2000).

2 The National Office of Statistics recorded a slight drop in the figures for 2006.

3 In *Leading Antenatal Classes* by Judy Priest and Judith Schott, 1991, Butterworth-Heinemann Ltd, 1991.

4 *Human Instinct*, presented by Professor Robert Winston, was first screened on BBC 1 in November 2002.

5 According to a report published by The Confidential Enquiries into Maternal Deaths (CEMACH) in 1997, more than half the 295 women who died during or after pregnancy between 2003 and 2005 were overweight or obese.

6 University of Texas researchers interviewed over 15,000 new mothers over 15 years and found a link between obesity at the time of conception and birth defects. Their findings are published in the journal Archives of *Pediatrics and Adolescent Medicine*.

7 According to an American report published in 2007 by the journal *Obstetrics & Gynecology* [sic].

8 According to a survey conducted by the children's charity Tommy's in 2007.

9 Grantly Dick-Read, *Childbirth Without Fear: The Principles and Practice of Natural Childbirth*, Pinter and Martin Ltd, July 2005 (First published by Harper in 1944).

10 Yehudi Gordon, *Birth And Beyond: Pregnancy, Birth, Your Baby and Family – The Definitive Guide*, 2002, Vermilion.

11 Motha and McGrath, *The Effects of Reflexology on Labour Outcome, Journal of Association of Reflexologists*: 2–4,1993.

12 Lewis E Mehl, MD, PhD, *Hypnosis and Conversion of Breech to Vertex Presentation*, from *Archives of Family Medicine*, Vol.3, Oct. 1994.

13 ME Hannah, WJ Hannah, The Term Breech Trial Collaborative Group 1997–2000.

14 BMJ editorial *How to Manage Term Breech Deliveries*, Andrew Shean and Susan Bewley, St Thomas's Hospital, London.

15 *The American Heritage Dictionary of English Language*, Fourth Edition, Copyright 2000 by Houghton Mifflin Company, updated in 2003.

16 According to the *Dr. Foster Good Birth Guide*, by Dr. Foster, Vermilion, 2005.

17 Roshni R Patel, Philip Steer, Pat Doyle, Mark P Little and Paul Elliot, *Does Gestation Vary By Ethnic Group? A London-based Study of Over 122,000 Pregnancies with Spontaneous Onset of Labour*, International Journal of Epidemiology 2003;33:107–113.

18 Cotzier wrote in the *British Medical Journal* in 1996 that 1 in 2000 babies were stillborn past 42 weeks gestation.

19 Cochrane review, Moore ER, Anderson GC, Bergman N., 2003.

20 Franco P et al, *Influence of Swaddling on Sleep And Arousal Characteristics of Healthy Infants, Paediatrics* Vol.115 No5 May 2005. Pp.1307-1311.

21 Dr De-Kun Li Kaiser and colleagues at Kaiser Permanente, California, and the National Institute of Child Health and Human Development, *Use of a Dummy (pacifier) During Sleep and Risk of Sudden Infant Death Syndrome (SIDS): Population Based Case-control Study, British Medical Journal* doi:10.1136/British Medical Journal.38671.640475.55, 9 December 2005.

22 Judith Lumley (1978), *Sexual Feelings in Pregnancy and After Childbirth, The Australian and New Zealand Journal of Obstetrics and Gynaecology* 18(2),114–117 doi:10.1111/j.1479–828X.1978.tb00026..X

resources

MEDICAL SERVICES

The National Institute of Clinical Excellence (NICE)
www.nice.org.uk

Finding a private obstetrician:
The Royal College of Obstetricians and Gynaecologists is the professional body for all doctors who specialize in this area.
www.rcog.org.uk

Finding an independent midwife:
www.independentmidwives.org.uk

SUPPORT AND INFORMATION

The Association for the Improvement of Maternity Services campaigns for a greater understanding of normal childbirth and for parents' rights within the maternity services.
www.aims.org.uk.
The children's charity Tommy's (www.tommys.org) offers lots of information about pregnancy.

Homebirth
www.homebirth.org.uk

SIDS
The Foundation for the Study of Infant Deaths (FSID)
www.fsid.org.uk
Stillbirth and Neonatal Society: 020 7436 5881
www.uk-sands.org

Down's syndrome
Down's Syndrome Association
www.downs-syndrome.org.uk

Antenatal testing
Antenatal Results and Choices (ARC Helpline: 020 7631 0285) provides non-directive support and information to parents throughout the antenatal

testing process. For information about invasive tests:
www.arc-uk.org/tests/screen.html
www.arc-uk.org/tests-explained

Small for dates/small for gestational age
Go to www.rcog.org.uk/index.asp?PageID=531 to download the pdf document entitled The Investigation and Management of the Small-for-Gestational-Age Fetus (31), November 2002 (a 'green-top' guideline).

Twins
The Multiple Births Foundation: 020 8383 3519
www.multiplebirths.org.uk and
www.twinsfoundation.com

Postnatal depression
The Association for Postnatal Illness: 020 7386 0868
www.apni.org

Depression/dealing with emotional issues
British Association for Counselling and Psychotherapy:
0870 443 5252
www.bacp.co.uk
Samaritans: 08457 909090, www.samaritans.org

Puerperal Psychosis
www.neuroscience.bham.ac.uk/research/app

For help quitting smoking
www.gosmokefree.co.uk

For help cutting down on alcohol
Drinkline: 0800 917 8282

For help with drug addiction
FRANK: 0800 776600. Counsellors on this information line are trained to help pregnant women with drug addictions.

Eating disorders
www.eating-disorders.org.uk
www.b-eat.co.uk

Domestic abuse
Free phone 24-hour National Domestic Violence
Helpline: 0808 2000 247
Victim Support: 0845 3030900
www.womensaid.org.uk
www.refuge.org.uk
For Legal Aid advisors:
www.communitylegaladvice.org.uk

Pre-eclampsia
www.pre-eclampsia.co.uk

Restless leg syndrome
www.rls.org

Obstetric cholestasis
www.ocsupport.org.uk

Miscarriage
www.miscarriageassociation.org.uk

Ectopic pregnancy
www.ectopic.org.uk

Incontinence
www.continence-foundation.org.uk

PARENTHOOD SUPPORT SERVICES

Support for mums
MAMA (Meet a Mum Association)
Helpline 0845 120 3746
www.mama.co.uk
The National Childbirth Trust
www.nctpregnancyandbabycare.com

Support for single mothers
www.gingerbread.org.uk

Information for working mums
For information on being pregnant at work see the
maternity section at *www.direct.gov.uk*
For information about pregnancy and employment
and your rights, see *www.direct.gov.uk*

Support and information for teenage mums
Connexions Direct: 080 80013219 text 07766413219
www.connexions.gov.uk

Support for dads
www.fathersdirect.com

Breastfeeding
La Leche League
Mother-to-mother support for and advice relating
to breastfeeding.
www.laleche.org.uk

Crying
Cry-sis: Helpline 020 7404 5011
www.cry-sis.org.uk
This helpline is open seven days a week for babies
with sleep problems.

Baby massage
Baby massage is taught throughout the UK. Contact
your local branch of the National Childbirth Trust for
details *www.nctpregnancyandbabycare.com*

Yoga with/for babies and children
There are lots of places that offer classes on yoga with
your baby. I particularly recommend YobaBugs.
www.yogabugs.com

Financial advice for parents
For information on child benefit and childcare
benefits, visit the Citizens Advice Bureau website at
www.adviceguide.org.uk and look under Your money –
Benefits, in the section entitled 'benefits for families
and children'.

HEALTH AND WELLBEING
DURING PREGNANCY

Healthy Start
The government initiative that provides free vitamins
and vouchers for milk, fresh fruit and vegetables.
www.healthystart.nhs.uk

Nutrition
www.foodforthebrain.org

Pregnancy yoga
Lolly Stirk, pregnancy yoga classes and birth preparation weekends/retreats, www.lollystirk.co.uk

Find a pregnancy Pilates class
www.pilatesfoundation.com
Nicki O'Clarey & Ramona Peoples: 07941 620 186
www.premierpilates.com
www.bodyorchestra.com
www.bodycontrol.co.uk

Find a reflexologist
www.findareflexologist.com
www.aor.org.uk
The Association of Reflexologists: 01823 351010
For information on essential oils and aromatherapy see www.aromatherapycouncil.co.uk

AIDS FOR LABOUR AND BIRTH

Doulas
Presently there are over 130 doulas registered in the UK. For information see: www.doula.org.uk

Swirls
www.jentlechildbirth.org.uk

TENS machine hire
www.tens.co.uk
www.mothercare.co.uk

Birthing balls
Try www.argos.co.uk

SPECIALIST PRODUCTS

The goi goi pillow
www.goigoibabypillows.co.uk

Elasticated button hooks
www.jojomamanbebe.co.uk

Lansinoh
Lansinoh is a topical salve specifically for cracked and painful nipples. See www.lansinoh.co.uk

Hypnobirthing CDs
Maggie Howell, natal hypnotherapy:
www.natalhypnotherapy.co.uk
The Hypnobirthing movement: www.hypnobirthing.co.uk
Gowri Motha: www.gentlebirthmethod.com

Pregnancy girdles
www.mothercare.co.uk
www.bumpsmaternity.com

SUGGESTED FURTHER READING

Michel Odent
This well renowned, pioneering obstetrician has written a number of books on different aspects of childbirth. Perhaps his best-known work is *Birth Reborn*, Souvenir Press Ltd, 1994.

Gowri Motha
Gentle Birth Method, Thorsons, 2004.

Ina May Gaskin
Spiritual Midwifery, Book Publishing Company (TN), 4th edition 2002, and *Ina May's Guide to Childbirth*, Bantam, 2003.

Penny Simkin
Comfort Measure for Childbirth, Childbirth Graphics, 1997. Fascinating information, in CD form.

Emma Mahony
For those expecting twins, I recommend *Double Trouble: Twins And How To Survive Them*, Thorsons, 2003. A funny and positive introduction to twins.

Marie Mongan
Hypnobirthing, Souvenir Press, 2007. Easy-to-follow techniques to help you achieve a peaceful birth.

index

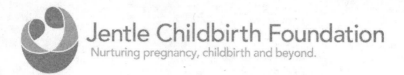

Jentle Childbirth Foundation

Nurturing pregnancy, childbirth and beyond.

The Jentle Childbirth Foundation is administered by the Institute of Obstetrics and Gynaecology Trust, registered charity 292518 (*www.iogt.org.uk*).

The Jentle Childbirth Foundation aims to:

• Create highly experienced and dedicated carers that can promote a safe, supportive and nurturing approach to birth.

• Explore and evaluate complimentary therapies and develop and distribute evidence-based models of care.

• Support a 'one-to-one' model of care, designed to allay the fear surrounding childbirth and to promote a positive experience for all women and their families.

Please see *www.jentlechildbirth.org*.uk for further details.

TO MAKE A DONATION

If you would like to help us further our aims and make a donation to the Jentle Childbirth Foundation, please do one of the following:

Go online at *www.jentlechildbirth.org.uk/donations* to pay by credit or debit card

or

Send your donation to Jenny Smith, c/o Gwen Young, IOGT, Wolfson and Weston Research Centre, Imperial College London, Hammersmith Hospital, Du Cane Road, London W12 0NN. Please make cheques payable to Institute Trust Fund and send us details of your name, address and indicate whether or not you are happy to Gift Aid your donation.

If you would like to discuss how you could help us further, please contact us on *nurturing@jentlechildbirth.org.uk*.